WHO SAYS I CAN'T

WHO SAYS I CAN'T

a two-time

cancer-surviving

amputee and entrepeneur

who fought back

survived

and thrived

JOTHY ROSENBERG

BASCOM
HILL BOOKS

Bascom Hill Books
212 3rd Avenue North, Suite 290
Minneapolis, MN 55401
612.455.2293
www.bascomhillpublishing.com

ISBN - 978-1-935456-13-1
ISBN - 1-935456-13-x
LCCN - 2009911465

Cover Design by Kristeen Wegner
Cover photo courtesy of The Boston Globe
Typeset by James Arneson

Printed in the United States of America

In memory of my niece Brianna,
a fighter to the end of her five-year life.

ACKNOWLEDGEMENTS

Arthur Graham is the prosthetist who builds and maintains my artificial leg. I have often thought he may have an inferiority complex about being as good as prosthetists who are also amputees. If that is the case, then his complex has resulted in spectacular achievement; he is better than any amputee prosthetist I have ever had. Whenever I go in for work on my leg (a "tune-up"), Arthur always wants to hear my stories, of which I have quite a few—many that make him laugh. He suggested I collect them into a book. And so began this memoir.

Jackie Herskovitz has been a friend since we met when I first started riding in the annual Pan-Massachusetts Challenge (PMC) bike-a-thon fundraiser. She leads PMC's public relations team and became a strong proponent of my efforts, my story, and this book. She was also an early reader with enthusiastic, but very honest, comments to improve the book.

Patrick McCoy has been a dear friend for thirty years. He presided as the minister over Carole's and my wedding. He was the sanest one in our group of three couples that formed the Smolka vacation group, later known as EPICS. Patrick was my spiritual counselor during my writing of this book. He helped me express myself in ways that would better reach people.

Zinta Aistars is a writer whom I have met only once. She wrote a wonderful article about me for the Kalamazoo College alumni magazine. She named that article "A Leg Up." Her questions and the resulting article were part of the process of motivating me to write this book. Zinta also introduced me to J. Conrad Guest, who made the first-pass edit and real contributions to the quality of this book.

Nicole Perrault, whom I have known for thirteen years, is a beautiful, smart, and delightful person. She ran a technical writing group for me when we first met and in three other jobs since, and she "knows writing." She is also a cancer survivor. She agreed to do a final edit pass before submission to the publisher. She is a joy to work with.

Erin Roof is a freelance journalist who moonlights as a book editor. She was commissioned by Bascom Hill Press to do the final edit on this book. I have never met Erin but she was a pleasure to work with. She is a meticulous editor who went above and beyond her commission because she really liked this project. The book is far better because of her efforts.

Jane Pince Acton is my oldest friend going back to seventh grade. She stuck with me at age sixteen when I lost my leg, and she was more crucial to me than any other friend ever was. We rarely see each other, but remain close. She assured the accuracy of my stories about those early years, and she made great suggestions to improve the book.

Joanna and Zac are my two youngest children. Along with Brendan, who is Carole's son from her previous marriage, my kids are the greatest highlights of my life. They are a constant positive reminder that I beat the odds. I not only survived, but also raised three amazing individuals in this world. Joanna and Zac tell me that I make them proud, and there are no words more positive that a parent could possibly hear. The feeling is mutual.

My wife, Carole, had two roles in this book. As always, she was extremely helpful with her sage wisdom and pragmatic advice, especially when it came to putting a more positive spin on some of my stories and checking for medical accuracy. She has also always been extremely encouraging of what I want or need to do, including writing this book. She took a huge chance on me. When she met me it was pretty well understood by the medical community that I might not be around for long. Since then, we have been through some rough times, but she always stuck with me. In recent birthday cards, she has said that I am an adventure and that I keep her young. Well, in return, she is my rock. She is the kindest, gentlest, most patient person I know, yet she still has a backbone of steel. I am extremely lucky. She is truly my soul mate.

PREFACE

One of the most difficult things everyone has to learn is that for your entire life you must keep fighting and adjusting if you hope to survive. No matter who you are or what your position is, you must keep fighting for whatever it is you desire to achieve.

—George Allen, football coach

"You have zero chance of survival." That is what my nineteen-year-old brain heard as my doctor told me that the cancer that took my right leg three years previously had now spread to my lung, two-fifths of which had also just been removed. What he probably said was, "No one has ever survived once this type of cancer spreads through the bloodstream." That was over thirty-five years ago. I survived. And then some.

This book is about what effect hearing those words has on someone's personality and how one can not only survive, but also fight back, recover, and thrive. This is not a "cancer book." Those are written when the survival is new and fresh and the experience is raw. Instead, this book, written with more than a thirty-five-year perspective, is about human perseverance, adaptability, and strength. People ask me all the time how my personality of today would be different had the cancer, amputation, loss of a lung, and death threat not occurred. I try to answer that in this book, but I do not believe anyone can say for sure what their personality would be like at age fifty if something had not happened to them at age sixteen or nineteen.

I am not famous and have not changed the world. But I have a story to tell, one that might help others. I was as devastated as one can possibly be after losing a leg at age sixteen, losing a major portion of a lung at age nineteen, having a year of chemotherapy, and all the while thinking I would die any day. I used athletics to redevelop self-confidence and became a double black diamond skier. I have ridden a bicycle, one-legged and one-lunged, from Boston to New York City three times, as well as 192 miles across Massachusetts seven times over a ten-year period to raise more than $100,000 for charity. I swim across San Francisco Bay every year in what is considered the most grand and intimidating competitive open water swims—also to raise money for charity. I have been married for more than twenty-eight years, adopted my wife's son, and had two more kids after Carole and I married, as well as one grandchild, all before I turned fifty. I earned a PhD in computer science, have written two technical books, and have started six high-technology companies, where I have been Chief Executive Officer, Chief Operating Officer, Chief Technology Officer, or Vice President. In starting those six companies, I raised more than $85 million in venture capital, with two of those companies providing a return of more than $100 million each. I could not have done all these startup companies if I had not developed the will power, determination, and focus that came from what happened to me, and if people had not kept saying, "I bet you can't," every place I turned.

Cancer is a devastating disease for sure. However, there are many other conditions that threaten people's lives and create some kind of disability: heart disease, diabetes, emphysema, cystic fibrosis, multiple sclerosis, and countless others. In the not-too-distant past, polio was the most dreaded disease; it disabled thousands. What polio survivors always seem to have in common is a drive to excel in the face of physical disability. Studies have compared them to the hard-driving, over-achieving individuals associated with Type A personality. In the words of one survivor, as captured by David M. Oshinsky in *Polio: An American Story*: "We were [taught] to be tough and gritty. I did what was expected. . . . I needed to have a disciplined life with a no-quit attitude. That was what worked." Lance Armstrong has said similar things about his cancer and how without his near-death experience and recovery he never would have gone on to win seven Tour de France races. I share these sentiments and feel that my experiences equipped me to tackle more and do better than I believe I would have otherwise.

There are 1.4 million new cases of cancer in the United States per year. There are 1.8 million Americans living with limb loss. There are 45 million disabled Americans. It is hard to imagine a single adult alive whose life has not been touched by cancer or disability. People who are knocked down by life need help and hope to fight back and win. Perhaps my story can provide a bit of that help and hope.

I cannot say that I have "cracked the code" on how to deal with adversity, the kind of adversity others have dealt with wonderfully well. However, many people over the years have told me that my story is inspirational to them. It took me a long time to look outside myself and my struggles and realize that I can motivate others around me. Maybe, with this book, I can shorten the recovery time for some people. I know I would have liked a book like this when I was a sixteen-year-old lying on my back in the hospital, wondering what—if anything—I would be able to do next and wondering how—if ever—I could be "normal."

I took the strength and fortitude I gained in fighting back from two bouts with cancer and a permanent disability and turned it toward business. High-tech startups are one of the toughest and riskiest flavors of business, yet I was drawn to them. So many things can go wrong in an early-stage startup. No startup I have heard of has ever realized success precisely according to plan. Change is inevitable and constant from the moment of formation. Being the leader of such risky ventures is by far the scariest and most challenging thing I have done in my professional life. I could not have kept going in the face of all the adversity I experienced starting six companies if not for the perspective I gained from surviving cancer and a permanent disability.

I have another message as well. I have endured a psychological adversity that has never gone away: the negative aspect of the word "considering." No one wants to hear, "You are good *considering*" in any circumstances. Whether it is because of gender, race, age, or a disability, "considering" neutralizes what would otherwise be a strong comment, a confidence builder—a compliment. "Considering" is a take-the-wind-out-of-your-sails word. It puts you in a different group, a separate-but-not-equal group. People with any sort of disability or disadvantage do not want to be part of that group. They work hard to be "normal." In fact, they have to work harder than the "normal" people whom they are trying to join. But the truth is, their disability actually gives them an edge. It makes them more focused, more disciplined, more determined. If their accomplishments are nullified with "considering," they are shoved right back into the unwanted realm of pity and sympathy. It crushes the confidence built up through all their hard work.

"Considering" is an insulting word. It demeans disabled people. It demeans minorities. It demeans children, women, ethnic groups, overweight people, the developmentally disabled, and on and on. I have heard the word all of my life. It has angered me and made me work harder. I have strived to ban it from any description of me, yet still I hear it.

Everyone falls into the trap and uses it, even friends. As in, "You ski pretty well . . . considering you have only one leg." "You sure throw a ball well . . . considering you are a girl." The examples are endless. "Great job you were offered . . . considering you are black." "You ran that mile pretty fast . . . considering you are only twelve." No one likes to deal with these put-downs, but the disabled can never escape them. The existence of the word "considering" should motivate us all to shatter the boundaries the world places on us.

When someone tempers your accomplishments with the word "considering" or rejects your aspirations with the phrase, "I bet you can't," the best defense is to show them that you can and you will. This book is about how I did just that and the insights with which I subsequently emerged. If these stories help just one person, I will have achieved my goal.

Within the limitations and frailties of human memory, I have tried to be accurate and factual in all incidents. In general, I have used people's actual names, but in some cases, names of people and companies have been changed to "protect the guilty."

Success is to be measured not so much by the position that one has reached in life as by the obstacles which one has overcome.

— Booker T. Washington, political leader

Jothy Rosenberg
Newton, Massachusetts, 2009

Part I — Double Jeopardy

dou•ble |ˈdəbəl| **jeop•ard•y** |ˈjepərdē|

noun. Risk or disadvantage incurred from two sources simultaneously[*]

---

*   Apple's OS X Dictionary

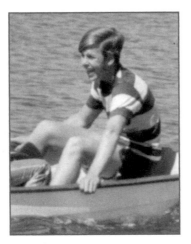

ONE

A MAVERICK TO REPLACE A LEG

The whole world loves a maverick.

— Kevin Patterson, author

The only disability in life is a bad attitude.

— Scott Hamilton, skater

Being defeated is often a temporary condition. Giving up is what makes it permanent.

— Marilyn vos Savant, journalist

It didn't seem like a life-changing event when it happened. It was October. I was sixteen, jumping rope in gym class at Wylie E. Groves High School in the Birmingham suburb of Detroit. While in midair, my right knee locked up as a searing pain shot up my leg, and I fell writhing to the cushioned mat. The class froze, sensing this was no minor injury. The pain was like nothing I had ever felt. It was blazing, sharp, and intense, focused in my knee, but with electric shock waves radiating up and down my entire leg if I moved it even a hair. After a while, I was able to get up with help, and the school called my parents to take me home.

Like always when we had medical issues, my father, a surgeon, was our primary physician. He examined me in our family room and saw no cause for alarm. "This is what happens to big, fast-growing boys who are very athletic," he said. "Your knee hurts. You fall. You twist a joint. It needs to be wrapped for support, and then you take it easy until it heals." That was the diagnosis. He expertly wrapped my knee in an ace bandage, and just as he had said, it improved a little each day.

Soon I was playing touch football, working in the yard, and running around our neighborhood. My strong, young body did a brilliant job of compensating for and adapting to what we did not know at the time: I had an extremely rare form of cancer that was destroying the healthy cells of the femur in my knee joint. The bone structure was disintegrating.

A few weeks later in November, at home in the yard, I was heading to the barn and needed to get over the paddock fence in a hurry. At the top of the fence, my knee locked up again. I fell, and it was even more painful this time than the incident in gym class.

I landed in a lump on the other side. It took a while before I could get up and limp back to the house. Dad wrapped it again and said I really had to take it easy this time to give it a chance to get better. I promised I would, and I meant it because this was getting to be a drag.

We had an amazing Golden Retriever named Lobo. He was officially my brother Michael's dog, but since Mike was off at college, Lobo became my constant companion. He was smart and well trained. I became the one who took him to a field for a run after school every day. I loved those runs. I was so proud of him, and he was a great substitute for not having any close high school friends since I had recently moved to a new school. I talked to him constantly while we wandered together through our favorite hiking area. He was so smart that I could just gently speak simple directions and he knew what I meant.

Christmas vacation came. On a wet, icy day in early winter, Lobo and I drove over to Franklin Village Green—a field about a mile from our house—for an afternoon walk. Although my knee was still wrapped, I was walking well, if a bit stiffly.

It was raining, and water was standing on the icy patches all over the Village Green, making it as slippery as a Teflon frying pan. Lobo blasted out of the car like a golden rocket. He was obedient to my voice commands, so I never leashed him. A proud, aggressive dog, he bounded through the field, sniffing and marking his territory. I opened my umbrella and followed him, gingerly traversing the slick ground.

Two hundred yards into the field, I hit an ice patch and my feet slipped out from under me. I must have looked like the cartoon character that slips and hangs suspended horizontally in midair before crashing to the ground. The pain from my previous falls didn't begin to compare to what I felt this time around. It was hard to breathe; I saw stars. It was raining and I had fallen into a puddle, which is probably all that kept me from going unconscious.

Lobo came right over and stayed by my side as I crawled and hopped back to the car. My right leg was useless, in excruciating pain. I struggled to lift it into the car and stay conscious. The car had a standard transmission, so I used the umbrella to press the accelerator and my left foot to work the clutch and brake. When I pulled into our driveway, I blasted the horn and kept blasting. The look on my father's face as he came running from the house took my breath away; it conveyed that he had—perhaps subconsciously—feared something like this might happen.

"Same knee," I managed to croak out when he asked me what had happened. "Hurts so bad. Can't walk."

No ace bandage this time. My parents mobilized into a flurry of activity to get me into the hospital for a biopsy that night. I suspect they (my mom especially, being a pathologist) had a feeling that it was bone cancer. But not wanting to worry me before they knew for sure, they didn't tell me anything. Being a sixteen-year-old, I assumed immortality. I did not think horrible things could possibly happen to me. Parents always worried too much, so I discounted their grim faces.

My father wrapped the knee tightly for the drive to the offices of Dr. Angelo Giambertoni, "Dr. G." I called him, in downtown Detroit.

Dr. G., Detroit's top orthopedist, quickly examined me. X-rays clearly showed the tumor and the irreparable damage the cancer had done to my knee. Still, my parents and Dr. G. needed to be certain.

On the short drive to Grace Hospital, my mother, a pathologist who specialized in tumors, explained that I needed a biopsy of the femur. "During the biopsy," she explained, "a long needle is inserted into the knee bone to take a very small sample of tissue for analysis so we will know for sure what's going on in there."

"You won't feel a thing," my father added. "You'll be under general anesthesia. It's quick, so you'll only be out for a short time."

The hospital quickly admitted me, and the nurses whisked me into surgery. I awoke to find my parents and Dr. G. hovering over me.

"I'm afraid we have some very bad news," said Dr. G. "The biopsy came back malignant, which means we have to amputate tomorrow at 7 a.m. Nurses will be here momentarily to begin prepping you for the surgery. Any questions?"

Malignant. Cancer. Amputation. Any questions? Was he kidding? I looked at my silent parents who couldn't make eye contact with me.

"It's just a sore knee from being a big active kid," I sputtered, throwing my dad's diagnosis back at them. "I promise to be more careful with it in the future."

I knew in my heart it was much more than that, but I wanted to buy time.

"The biopsy is definitive," Dr. G. continued. "It reveals the presence of a type of bone cancer called 'osteogenic sarcoma' in the femur side of your knee. We have to take your leg off above the knee to get the cancer out, and we have to move quickly so the cancer cells don't enter your blood stream and spread."

In my simplified view of the world, smoking caused cancer. It afflicted old people. How could it be inside *me*? And Dr. G. wanted to cut off my leg! I was beyond petrified. Dr. G. was waiting for my consent before he put the staff in motion to prep me for surgery.

"I'm not letting you take my leg unless my mom tells me there is no alternative," I said.

My mother would realize my condition was not all that serious when she looked at the biopsy. I had total faith in her. Over the years, I had heard her colleagues gush about what a rock star doc she was.

It may seem cruel and self-centered to have involved my mother, but anyone going through the kind of ordeal I went through should be allowed to be selfish at times. The newly disabled, those diagnosed with life-threatening illnesses, and those who have suffered a tremendous loss, need time within themselves to recover psychologically. That kind of self-centeredness is crucial in order to reclaim your life. If you don't focus on yourself, you may not find the inner strength you need to fight back.

In *Lucky Man: A Memoir*, Michael J. Fox writes about his reaction to his Parkinson's diagnosis: "Nobody would ever choose to have this visited upon them. Still, this unexpected crisis forced a fundamental life decision: adopt a siege mentality—or embark upon a journey."

A journey is a wonderful way to view life after a diagnosis like Fox's or mine. At sixteen, however, there was no way I had that level of maturity. It was only years later, many years into adulthood, that I was able to see that my diagnosis was actually the beginning of a journey toward the meaning and purpose of my life. A journey we all have to take, disabled or not.

My mother obtained permission to look at my biopsy tissue, although I was not officially her case. I waited anxiously for her return, hoping she would spare me.

Mom had a commanding presence, thin and standing six feet tall. She was stoic—a reserved New Englander who rarely showed emotion. I had never so much as seen her shed a tear, but when she returned to my room, she was pale and trembling. She stood next to my hospital bed, and I will never forget her words. "Jothy," she said, "there is no choice but to amputate your leg."

My father, typically a pillar of strength, was also on the verge of tears. Seeing them struggle to keep their composure terrified me. I began to weep, and at that point, they couldn't hold back their tears any longer.

I eventually regained enough composure to give Dr. G. my formal consent to amputate my leg.

My mother reiterated that the cancer could get into the blood stream and latch on somewhere else, which is why the surgery had to happen immediately. I assumed the chance that the cancer had entered my bloodstream was remote and that they just liked covering their bases no matter how unlikely the scenario. Little did I know.

I would later learn that my type of bone cancer, osteogenic sarcoma, now more commonly known as "osteosarcoma," strikes only nine hundred people in the United States each year, almost all of them children. It is fifty percent more likely to occur in boys than girls, possibly because it may be related to rapid bone growth. It is deadly. If the cancer cells get into the blood stream, they like to metastasize to new sites. Metastasize means to spread from one part of the body to another. When cancer cells metastasize and form secondary tumors, the cells in the metastatic tumor (called "mets") are like those in the original (primary) tumor. With many types of cancers, the most common site for mets is the lungs, which are the first place cells land after venous blood returns to the heart.

In 1973, when this particular cancer metastasized to a lung, it was a death sentence. My physician parents both knew this. As they looked down at their weeping son, I now understand that they saw not just the loss of a leg, but also the potential loss of their child.

Early the next morning, a busy dance of nurses, orderlies, and doctors began. My parents, who exuded an overwhelming sense of sadness, had to stay out of the way. I was on strong pain meds, sedated to blunt the inevitable terror of what was coming. They put me on a gurney and wheeled me to the operating room. Someone placed a mask over my mouth and told me to count backwards from ten. I was out by the time I got to five.

As I began to regain consciousness from the deep fog of anesthesia, I found myself in a dark, quiet recovery room. All I could see were curtains near my bed and some nurses studying monitors and papers on their desks just across from where I was lying. All I could hear were machines making quiet, high-tech whirring and beeping noises. I knew what was supposed to have happened, so I looked down. It was gone. A large bandaged stump was all that was left of my right leg. The anesthesia numbed my shock and horror of that first sighting, but an overwhelming sense of loss and sadness settled over me. Although my brain was too foggy to crisply analyze the situation, the nurses focused me on practical matters right away. Unless I could pee on my own, they threatened, they would insert a catheter to drain my bladder. Two sets of strong arms stood me up on my one leg. I was weak and dizzy, but finally the urine came.

Peeing on my own was actually a critical first step. *At least*, I thought, *I have been able to accomplish that.* It was something on which to build a return to a normal life.

I desperately wanted to be normal. For a new amputee, normalcy is an elusive dream. It is like grabbing for the Crisco-covered watermelon in the pool games I played at summer camp. You can see the watermelon. You can almost touch it. But then, as soon as you grab hold of it, it squirts away and you have to chase after it all over again.

The feeling of being normal is especially important to the child or teenage amputee. Being part of the group and able to do what the rest of the kids are doing is vital. But sports, dancing, and dating seemed completely out of reach for someone looking down at a stump where his leg once was.

As I was grappling with my new body, trying to pee, and dealing with the horrible feeling in my gut that I would never again fit in, I also had to face the fact that the amputation had not gone well.

As it turned out, Dr. G. usually did amputations on elderly patients with poor circulation and weak muscles. He was unfamiliar with strong, young legs with normal blood flow, and, because of that, he had almost lost me on the operating table.

In elderly people with poor circulation, a tourniquet placed above the cut line for the amputation is sufficient to stop any bleeding. For a leg with healthy musculature and vasculature, however, the recommended technique is to cut toward the bone, tie off all the major blood vessels, and then cut a little deeper. This procedure is much more time consuming than using a tourniquet, which may have been one of the reasons Dr. G. elected not to use it.

As Dr. G. must have quickly discovered, however, it is difficult to secure the air-filled tourniquet around well-toned muscles. Worse, because one's thigh narrows as it gets closer to the knee, the tourniquet has a tendency to slip downward. When that happens, the tourniquet loosens, taking pressure off the deeper arteries in the lower leg. It is still tight enough, however, to occlude the venous return vessels that are closer to the surface. That, in turn, raises the pressure in the arteries, causing them to bleed even more profusely.

The old rule of thumb when doing an amputation for bone cancer was to make sure there was a joint between the amputation site and the cancerous bone. That would have meant cutting my leg off at the hip. Wearing a prosthesis with no stump at all is problematic, so Dr. G. elected to leave me with part of my thigh, but still cut high enough up the leg to put some distance between the cut point and the tumor. When the tourniquet slipped and the bleeding increased, I was continuously transfused as Dr. G. raced to finish the amputation. On the table, I bled out six of my sixteen units of blood and ended up with a five-inch stump, which is way too short to work well with a prosthesis.

To make matters worse, Dr. G. bent my leg at the hip so it would be easier to work on. Imagine lying flat on your back with your legs straight out. If Dr. G. had amputated in that position, my stump would have lined up with my upper body and left leg. But he bent my right leg, flexing the hip, and removed it midway between the hip and knee as he tied off all the muscles. That bend in my hip became permanent, and it has been a nightmare for me ever since. In the language of amputees, this is called "flexion contracture." The muscles in the front of my leg are tied off shorter than the muscles in back, and no amount of physical therapy or stretching can ever make my residual limb (or stump) stay straight, which makes fitting a prosthesis exceedingly difficult.

Giambertoni's decision to cut so far up the leg was also a bad one. Every millimeter of residual limb becomes vitally important for leverage inside the socket of an artificial leg. The more leverage, the more control. The more control, the less limping. My short, flexed stump has given me a pronounced, unavoidable, and permanent limp.

I wish I could tell you this was the extent of my challenges, but the extreme blood loss and excessive tourniquet tightness, and a fight against time to finish the amputation, caused an unusually high degree of tissue trauma, massive swelling, and bleeding—all of which contributed, post surgery, to horrific phantom pain.

Calling pain "phantom" makes it sound unreal. Let me assure you, that is not at all the case. It is a cruel joke at the expense of the amputee. Fifty to eighty percent of the roughly two million amputees in the United States feel as though they have pain coming from a body part that no longer exists.

American military surgeon Silas Weir Mitchell first coined the term "phantom limb" in 1871. It was much earlier, in 1551, that the French military surgeon Ambroise Paré wrote, "For the patients, long after the amputation . . . say that they still feel pain in the amputated part." Until recently, many believed this post-amputation phenomenon was a psychological problem. Amputees were told that if they felt pain in a missing limb, they had mental problems and should see a psychiatrist.

It was not until the early 1970s that researchers learned from brain mapping that the nerves firing in the residual limb after an amputation are transmitted to the somatosensory cortex, the part of the brain responsible for the movement and exchange of sensory and motor information, including pain. The pain amputees feel from these traumatized nerves is just as real as the pain you feel when you cut your finger with a knife.

The part of the somatosensory cortex responsible for phantom sensation is similar to a hard-wired telephone switchboard, with a plug for every nerve coming from the body's surface. This area is not part of the conscious brain, and it does not know where its signals originate. A signal from a nerve on the stump that once extended all the way to the foot is routed through the somatosensory cortex, which tells the conscious brain there is a sensation in the foot. The conscious brain, which knows full well that the foot is gone, is powerless to override these signals.

Phantom pain can feel like burning, stinging, or worst of all, shooting electric shocks. It is worse in people who experience pain before or right after their amputation. It is now recognized that pain management in both cases is critical. Jonathan Cole at The Wellcome Trust, who has studied phantom pain extensively, describes it as "often excruciating and almost impossible to treat," adding that it can be "intractable and chronic."[*]

In my case, the phantom phenomenon, pain included, has turned out to be permanent. Even thirty-six years after my amputation, I can still try to wiggle my non-existent toes. My stump aches and tingles, sometimes severely, almost every night, which makes me a poor sleeper. Sometimes waves of what feel like high-voltage electric shocks shoot through my body, reminding me (as if I needed reminding) of the trauma of my operation. Occasionally, these debilitating waves can last an entire day, completely taking me out of commission. There is no rhyme or reason to when a bad day is going to occur. Psychologically, phantom pain drains you; you feel like you already "paid the price," and yet the pain never lets up. You keep paying and paying. Sometimes it makes you want to scream. Or cry.

Once I came out of anesthesia, I needed morphine, but I was given Demerol. In 1973, the medical community feared putting patients on narcotics would turn them into drug addicts. I was sure glad when my father changed the orders on my chart, even if it may have violated medical protocol. On Demerol, I had been sluggish, cloudy, dazed, and still in agonizing pain. On morphine, I was clear-headed, sharp-witted, and the pain was almost gone. It is now generally accepted in the medical community that narcotics administered for pain for a short time, especially when self-administered, do not cause addiction.

---

[*]   Cole, Jonathan, *Phantom Limb Pain*, http://www.wellcome.ac.uk/en/
    pain/mcrosite/medicine2.html

The hospital staff stood me on one leg so I could start relearning balance and be able to pee without support. But as hard as I tried, I could not remain upright without my crutches. My body and brain played tricks on each other. My brain remembered how balance felt before the amputation, when I had stood on one leg while I still had the other leg to move around as a counterbalance. It sent the same signals as it always had to the muscles in both my legs. The muscles on the left side did as they were told. On my right side, however, there were no muscles to receive my brain's signals. As I tilted to one side, my inner ear became unbalanced and sent that signal to the brain, which would futilely try to get my missing right leg to do its part to regain my balance. Fortunately, the brain relearns quickly and within weeks I was balancing unconsciously again.

I had the weird idea when I began to think more clearly that they should weigh the amputated leg. I wanted to be able to quote an extrapolated weight. They reported my limb weighed twenty-five pounds. Today, when someone asks me how much I weigh, I have to figure from three different possible answers. My as-is, no-clothing, one-legged, six feet two inch weight is 185 pounds. My two-legged, *extrapolated* weight is 210 pounds, which more closely resembles what people think when they see me. My weight wearing my prosthesis is 197 pounds. The one I usually quote to avoid confusion is the extrapolated, guesstimate weight.

As I began to recover, I started asking questions. When would I get a prosthesis? How long would it take to relearn how to walk? Would I be able to ski? Ice skate? No one could give me answers.

When I told my first joke, which was silly and a little morbid, people acted as though it was a huge deal. "You finally found a cure for the athlete's foot problem I had on my right foot," I quipped. It was a sign that I was rediscovering my personality and doing what I always did: trying to make light of whatever it was that was stressing me. I was emerging from the fog of self-pity and beginning to deal with what had happened.

Stephen Hawking, the world famous physicist and bestselling author who, at age twenty, was diagnosed with Amyotrophic Lateral Sclerosis (also referred to as "Lou Gehrig's Disease"), has spent almost fifty years in a wheelchair. He spoke frequently about the attitude that has sustained him. "It is a waste of time to be angry about my disability," Hawking said in a 2005 interview with *The Guardian* newspaper. "One has to get on with life, and I haven't done badly. People won't have time for you if you are always angry or complaining."

Hawking and everyone else who has faced a limiting physical condition knows how easy it is to slip into self-pity. We are all prone to it, disabled or not. We would all do well to listen to people like Hawking, for whom self-pity is anathema. The definition of *self-pity* in Merriam-Webster's online dictionary is "a self-indulgent dwelling on one's own sorrows or misfortunes."

Regaining confidence is where our personal fight begins. It's rare to find a person—able-bodied or disabled, healthy or sick—who has not been knocked down by life at one time or another. Regaining confidence is particularly difficult when we face a debilitating physical challenge, but we need to transcend our human propensity for self-pity if we want to feel fully alive and live up to our potential.

I've always found that my confidence is boosted when I push my body to the limit—skiing, riding my bike, swimming long distances—and deal with the physical pain. Win one victory; go on to the next battle; and win that too. Pretty soon, these little victories start to add up to confidence. At that point, self-pity becomes but a distant memory.

It was depressing to me then, but looking back now, it's just plain shocking that one and only one friend had the guts to visit me in the hospital. Jane Pince was a friend from junior high that went to the high school across town. She visited me several times in the hospital and then at the house before I was able to go back to school. Teenagers are self-focused and afraid of illness in others, but Jane still recognized that when something this devastating happens, the victim needs support and friendship more than ever. When I talk to teenagers now about disability, I make a specific point to challenge them: what would you do if your friend got whacked like that and was in the hospital? I hope that times have changed and the teenagers of today would behave differently than the teenagers of 1973.

As it turned out, I spent only five days in the hospital. During that time, I began to develop an attitude that has sustained me through my life. When the doctors said I would need to stay in the hospital for two weeks, I took it as a challenge to beat their estimate. *"Who says I can't be ready in one?"* I asked myself. It was the first of many times I would sound my new rallying cry.

Glad as I was to leave Grace Hospital behind, the real world felt like a strange and scary place in which I no longer belonged. I had absolutely no idea how I was going to cope as I looked out the window of our station wagon on the ride home.

As we pulled into the driveway, there was a green Ford Maverick with a ribbon around it. I immediately knew it was for me. What sixteen-year-old boy, even if he had lost his leg only five days before, wouldn't jump (dare I say hop) for joy at the sight? Tears welled up in my parent's eyes as they acknowledged my excitement and appreciation. It was the first of many examples of how they intuited just the right amount of help to provide, balanced with an equal amount of challenge, to make me stretch and grow.

Even the Maverick couldn't take away the pain, however, once I was back home, off morphine, and relying solely on codeine. The pain was intense, sharp, and throbbing. There was no relief. I couldn't sleep, watch television, read, or even carry on a conversation.

I tried not to look at the stump when my dad changed my dressings once a day. I did see, however, that there was a giant incision across the end of what was left of my leg. It was red, bruised, swollen to twice its normal size, and crisscrossed with stitches. It frightened and appalled me, and I couldn't accept that it was part of me and would be for the rest of my life.

Looking down at myself, I was beginning to become accustomed to seeing my right leg missing. But I hated looking at myself in the mirror; reflected back at me, the difference in my body was extreme. I felt like a freak.

I slept fitfully for short durations. The pain always seemed worse at night. I would lie in bed, unbearably lonely, crushed by the searing waves of pain, acutely aware of my deformed body, cursing my fate, and asking myself over and over, "Why me?"

Music was an escape from the nightmare of my new body. My method of escapism could have been much more extreme. Believe me, I know how strong the temptation is to use drugs to blunt the pain and anxiety of a life that has been severely compromised. I was lucky to be able to lose myself instead in "Locomotive Breath" by Jethro Tull, "Riders on the Storm" by The Doors, "Stairway to Heaven" and "Kashmir" by Led Zeppelin, and "In the Court of the Crimson King" by King Crimson. I listened to the albums with those songs over and over. When I hear that music today, it still evokes powerful feelings of healing and recovery.

Chronic pain is much better understood now than it was then. But even in the early 1970s, it was known that a "cognitive busy signal" could be created in the brain to block or suppress the sensation of pain. Intense focus on a task can create this kind of busy signal. Solitaire, puzzles, models, and building a stereo from a kit created the busy signals I needed and kept me focused.

True to form, I pushed and pushed, and my parents and doctors finally relented and let me go back to school after just three weeks at home—five weeks less than the eight they had told me I would have to endure. I wanted to go back to school not only to begin leading a normal life again, but also to smash through the limits being placed on me and to exceed everyone's expectations. When they said, "you can't," I was determined to show them I could. I would beat their predictions if it killed me.

I went back to school on crutches. In those days, they waited six months between amputation and fitting an artificial leg to allow complete muscle atrophy and de-swelling of all the soft tissues in the stump. Today it's different. A new amputee is immediately fitted with a prosthesis because it actually helps decrease the swelling of the stump by placing it snugly inside a hard plastic socket. This also gives the amputee a head start on the challenge of relearning to walk.

Groves High was an E-shaped building with 2,100 students in three grades. The spine of the E was the main hall from which feeder halls branched. Between classes, the main hall was packed with kids at their lockers, talking in groups, and coupling up. It was a loud, busy place. But not on my first day back. When I swung through on crutches, it was like the parting of the Red Sea.

While I had been in the hospital, there had been a detailed public address announcement about my plight. All Groves' 2,100 students—most of whom had no idea who I was—now knew the tragic story of the one-legged guy in their midst. They jumped out of my way as I approached, became suddenly quiet, and gawked. No one talked to me. No one even made eye contact.

I felt their pity and discomfort—it was sickeningly thick in the air—as I focused with all my might on trying not to stumble. Their pity infuriated me. It forced me away from them, away from their healthy, two-legged, mobile, athletic lives. I felt isolated, freakish, and singled out. I was still me, but I felt utterly and completely defined by my missing leg.

The anger I felt at people's pity and my determination to defy expectations spurred me to become a wiz on crutches. I refused to let people hold doors for me. Instead, I figured out how to smash school-building horizontal bar openers with my foot. I came at a door full speed, pivoting back and balancing on my crutches so that my one leg was almost horizontal with my hips, and fired my foot into the bar. The door flew open and I swung on through. Luckily, no one was ever opening the door from the other side at the same time. But I was not really thinking too much about other people. It was all about me and about counteracting the horrible feelings of pity I felt from all sides. I was angry and scared, and I had a big chip on my shoulder.

My body began to adapt to its new form. My balance improved. Walking on crutches is essentially walking on your arms, and my arms and remaining leg naturally grew stronger.

I cruised along at a good clip. Stairs slowed me down, so I invented special stair adaptations. Going up, I took stairs two at a time, leading with my foot and following with the crutches. I went down even faster. After taking two steps down, leading with the crutches, I landed on the same step as the crutches with my foot; a little hop and a slide off the edge of that step got me down one extra step, while the crutches moved down two more steps. So it was two steps plus one extra each cycle—a very fast stair descent indeed. Incredible as it may seem, in thirty-six years of doing this I have never fallen.

The doctors were probably right: it was a bit early to be back in school. I was anemic from blood loss, tired, and unable to concentrate in class. The phantom pain was severe. Fortunately, the school let me come and go as I pleased. The Maverick made that easy. What mattered to me was that I was back much earlier than anyone had thought possible. Who said I couldn't? Just winning that battle alone gave me confidence.

I had lost a leg during my Christmas vacation, but that winter I began to find ways to fight back from what felt like a complete and crushing defeat. I had no idea what was in front of me, and I often fell back into feelings of self-pity and despair. I was angry much of the time, and I felt very much on my own. I began to set goals and work hard at them.

I celebrated even the smallest victories. Smashing open doors. Going up and down stairs. Relearning to drive. Taking Lobo for a hike on crutches. Each one of those little things felt like a fight to me because I was being constantly tested, knocked down, and pushed up against my limitations. I was in constant pain and struggling to learn how to live with that pain and accept my new body. And I was beginning to find a new way to move through the world—the way of the amputee, the disabled, the cancer survivor.

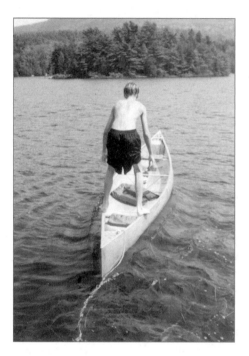

WILL POWER

Stubbornness is also determination. It's simply a matter of shifting from "won't power" to "will power."

— Peter McWilliams, author

You gain strength, courage, and confidence by every experience in which you really stop to look fear in the face. You are able to say to yourself, I have lived through this horror. I can take the next thing that comes along. . . . You must do the thing you think you cannot do.

— Eleanor Roosevelt, former first lady

Six months after my amputation, I was fitted for an artificial leg—a prosthesis. A "wooden leg," literally. Except for the metal knee joint and the plastic foot, it was all balsa wood; it was very light, but still strong. It fastened to my stump with suction. The top of the prosthesis was formed into a socket, custom-fitted to my stump. I used a sock to pull the stump into this tight-fitting socket through a small hole in the socket's bottom. After I pulled the sock through the hole, a twist of a one-way valve screwed into the hole let out any air bubbles and prevented air from leaking back in through the valve. When I was done with the sock, I flipped it over my shoulder for a moment. Often I forgot it was there and endured many an embarrassing moment when someone noticed a little lump on my shoulder under my shirt.

Learning how to walk with one of these contraptions takes at least six months. Humans have sensors in their flesh and blood joints called "proprioceptors" that tell them, even when they are not looking, what positions their limbs are in. As an amputee, because the joint is gone, so are the proprioceptors. I had to use another sense, like sight, to know where the artificial foot was. This is extremely critical because if I happened to step on the leg when the knee was bent, I quickly learned how fast gravity works. Unfortunately, this was a lesson I have ignominiously learned repeatedly throughout my one-legged life. The average amputee falls several times a week.

In the early days, the knees swung freely when they were initially unweighted, as the prosthesis' toe came off the ground from behind. Once the leg swung all the way forward, it was ready to bear weight. And once the heel struck the ground in front of the amputee, and his knee was weighted, it locked in place to support him as he put full weight on it, ready to unweight his real leg. At first, a new amputee must look down to see when the heel hits the ground and the knee is straight so he knows it will hold him. Later he will know by timing when he can put weight on the leg.

I eased into walking with the prosthesis using two crutches. After two months, I went to one crutch. Eventually, and this step was hard, I moved to a cane. I ended up using a cane for three more years, all through college, until I finally pitched it away with some dramatic flair.

In the quest for normalcy, getting the prosthesis was a major step. But it was a double-edged sword. I walked with a limp, but I looked like I had two legs, and maybe just a bum knee. I could carry things, like a plate at a buffet dinner or grocery bags on a shopping trip. Or a baby. I stopped being stared at everywhere I went. This was all good and a wonderful confidence builder, but there are glitches with a prosthesis. Each glitch, no matter how many years have gone by, can shatter my confidence and sense of normalcy. In the course of minutes, I can go from feeling happy to help by running to the store for a loaf of bread or a carton of milk, to feeling literally crippled and not wanting to go anywhere. All it takes is stepping on a marble or a LEGO and taking a tumble. Or maybe the leg fit has changed, making me wince in agony with every step, or the knee is unstable because it needs a minor readjustment. Early on, my expectations were so low that it was hard for the leg to disappoint me. But it grew to be a part of me that I needed to depend on—to trust—and it has not always come through.

I have never wanted a first meeting with someone when I was not wearing my prosthesis; it created a difference. Any difference creates the perception of an imbalance. This is the real point of prosthetics—to level the playing field of interpersonal dynamics so the disabled individual can focus on the *normalcy* of social interactions without worrying about the "rhinoceros in the room."

Dad sensed correctly that I needed a major push to get me to learn how to use the prosthesis. He thought a job that required strength and mobility was just the thing for me that first summer with my new leg. I would be acclimating to the prosthesis, while doing something productive that would make me feel useful again. Using his connections, he got me a job at the local VA hospital pushing the 400-pound food trucks from the kitchen up to the patient floors for each meal, and later bringing them back down to the kitchen for cleaning and the next meal. The truck acted as my cane while I pushed it, and so I placed my real cane across the top of the truck until I needed it to get back down to the kitchen to get another truck. Each day at the end of my shift, my stump would bleed from the wear and tear on my skin. But I could see progress in my walking, and my overall strength began to build.

I wanted to be able to do whatever two-legged people could do. I still took my dog Lobo on a hike every day, but not with my leg. An artificial leg is probably like a tight dress shoe. It's the kind of thing one wears when necessary, but it's quick to come off when it's time to relax or do anything athletic.

This is especially true for an above-knee amputee and doubly so for one with a stump as short as mine. The leg wielded a lot of leverage on my hip, so I never wanted to be in a sport with it on. Without a knee, it offered no help in skiing, biking, or hiking, and, of course, it would be dead weight (and be ruined) when swimming. When it came off, it stood in the corner of the room by my bed. My pants stayed on it, as did the sock and shoe. The next day I might not need to change the pants, and since socks smell only from sweaty feet and my foot was plastic, it could stay on a really long time. The only problem was making sure my socks matched when picking a mate from the sock drawer. Frequently I guessed wrong. There were even times—I wish I could say infrequently— when I would have one dark sock and one white sock. Eventually, I decided that matching socks just weren't a priority. That stopped working once my daughter was old enough to check and send me back upstairs to change when I got it wrong.

When taking Lobo on long hikes in the woods, the prosthesis was beyond useless because of the uneven ground. Crutch walking was building up my arm strength as well as that of my real leg. I used the full-length crutches for better stability. All my weight was always on my hands. This meant a hike for me was much more work and a better workout than the same hike for two-leggers.

My family got very tired of saying "prosthesis," or "artificial leg," so they decided it needed a nice friendly name. Besides, it seemed to have a personality, complete with a strange sense of humor, all its own. So they named it "Herbie." I liked that name so it stuck. Herbie started to have some interesting adventures.

My brother Michael's girlfriend, Vicki (whom he would eventually marry), was pretty volatile. And, like a typical seventeen-year-old, I loved pushing her buttons. One morning I came up to breakfast and she was at the table. For no particular reason other than I was a bratty teenager feeling my oats, I started teasing her and went too far. Suddenly she stood up, turned toward me, wound up her leg, and kicked me with all her might. She used her left leg, however, which meant she hit me on my right side—the side made out of very hard wood and plastic. Her anklebone lost that particular fight. At first, I was shocked that she had kicked me. My shock turned to wonderment that I had felt absolutely nothing, and then it quickly devolved into uncontrollable laughter. I was exceedingly lucky that Vicki had forgotten which side of me was "real" and hadn't kicked the other side—or worse, halfway in between. To this day, she has a little bone spur on her ankle to remind her of her temper and the futility of trying to kick her hard-like-a-rock brother-in-law.

I had always liked doing yard work, and because we had a riding mower, I was able to get right back to doing that job. I would leave the crutches in the storage shed and drive out on the tractor after making sure it was full of gas. I could do the entire two-acre grassy part of the yard in a couple of hours on a full tank. It was therapeutic. It was liberating. I was doing something useful, and I thoroughly enjoyed it. Except once.

My younger brother had several unorthodox hobbies for a twelve-year-old boy. He knitted, rode horses, and kept bees; later, he became a lawyer, a businessman, and a father. The beehive sat on the grass down by the horse paddock, well away from the house. As most bees are, I suppose, these bees were very protective of their hive, especially on one hot August afternoon. Whenever I went around the beehive boxes on the riding mower, I kept them on my left so the forced air coming out of the mower on the right didn't blow toward the bees. On that particular day, for some reason, I forgot. Just as I came around the white hive boxes—with them on my right—I had three thoughts. First, I marveled at the number of bees cooling themselves out on the front of the hive.

Second, I thought *Oh shit* as I realized I was going the wrong way around the hive, but it was too late. The strong wind and grass from the mower blew the thousands of bees, innocently minding their own business, off the front of the hive. It looked like I had thrown a basket of black beads directly into a powerful fan. At first, they sailed toward the fan, but then they all turned to head back from where they came. Toward me. Unlike a bucket of black beads, those little nasties all had stingers and minds of their own. And they were majorly pissed off. Time for my third thought: *Run. Oops. Can't do that. Okay then. Hop!* I left the tractor motor running, got off, and hopped as fast as my one leg would go toward the tool shed. The hives were way up at the front of the two-acre yard and the shed was at the back of the yard. I hopped more than one hundred yards. I couldn't believe how fast I could hop with thousands of bees after me. Bees hit me and got into my hair and down my shirt. Many stung me, so I waved and slapped my hands furiously as I madly hopped across the yard to escape their much-deserved wrath. By the time I made it to the shed and got any last lingerers off me, I had been stung dozens of times. If only Guinness had been there, I could have been in their book of records for one-legged hopping speed and distance. Of course, the tractor was still running way down there by the hives and I had to go back down to it. But once things calmed down, I could do that in a bit more dignified manner on crutches. I never again violated the "only pass their hives with them on your left" rule. My brother was most upset that all the bees that stung me had died and would no longer be able to make honey or more baby bees. I gave him a small, brotherly attitude adjustment for that comment.

It took a long time, but finally, in my senior year of high school, I got up the nerve to date. I was getting the hang of the prosthesis and starting to feel like I could recover some semblance of normal high school life. Most importantly, the prosthesis allowed me to remove that sense of pity I believed—true or not—I felt from girls.

In our family, whenever any of us kids were out at night—date or no date—we had a strict curfew time of 11 or 11:30. We needed to be accurate to the minute or the consequences were severe. When we reached high school age, Dad used a trick to check if we were drunk or stoned when we arrived home late. He taught us all a rhyme that we had to recite. If we could say it correctly without slurring our words, we were off the hook. If we could not, we were punished. The rhyme is burned into my brain cells. In fact, I think I can recite it when drunk to this day. It goes like this:

One fat hen,
Two ducks,
Three cackling geese,
Four plump partridges,
Five pairs of Don Alfonzo tweezers,
Six limerick oysters,
Seven sympathetic apathetic didactic
    old gentlemen on crutches,
Eight hundred Macedonian Horseman
    drawn up in full battle array,
Nine crates of withered Monkeys
    drawn from the sepulchers of ancient Egypt,
Ten heliospheric gold beads
    procured for the Armesyrian Institute.

Sara Hulse was the driving motivation for dating. I was completely enamored with her. She was tall, athletic, blond, and beautiful. She was nice, and she was smart. Actually going through with a date was a huge deal for me, but I took the plunge and asked Sara to go to *Tommy*, The Who's rock opera movie. Both Sara and I had to use the restrooms before the movie. As I left the sink on the way out, Herbie's foot caught on a little rug. I felt the tug of my right foot as I kept walking, but I pulled hard to free it and luckily did not fall in the process. But when my "foot" came down on the next step, I landed on nothing but a bare bolt. No foot. I looked at the rug, now behind me, and saw with horror my foot, with a sheared off bolt sticking out of it, caught on the curled up part of the rug. I reached down and grabbed the foot and hopped out the door and over to the benches right outside the bathroom. I was stunned. I just sat there holding the foot out in front of me staring at it. Of course, now I was worried about how I would get into and out of the movie. In the back of my mind, I also knew that my great hopes of getting lucky with Sara that night were dashed.

This was 1974 and *Tommy* was the kind of movie that many kids went to see stoned. Guys with bloodshot eyes and smoke swirling around them gave me wild stares as they came out of the rest room. As I gaped at the foot I was still holding in front of me, one of them said to me, "Wow, man, did that hurt?" That helped bring me out of my momentary despair, and I began to see the humor in the situation. Then Sara came out and, without missing a beat, asked what she should do to reattach my foot. I did not need to answer; she immediately figured out what I needed. She got a roll of masking tape from the concession counter. (Duct tape would have been much better and things might have turned out differently.) She had me put the foot up against her shoulder, with the rest of the leg lined up correctly, while she created a new ankle out of masking tape. She went round and round using the entire roll of tape, creating a nice fat tape ankle.

I could now shuffle my way into the movie using Sara as a cane on my left side. I didn't really enjoy the movie very much, as I worried the whole time about getting back to the car and beyond. The shuffle out to the car ended up disintegrating this fine ankle. It rained while we were in the theatre, and unavoidable puddles caused the masking tape to dissolve, but I was able to make it to the car. I took Sara home, but stayed in the car to drop her off. Not the suave moves I had been planning and practicing for weeks. It was a disappointing evening, but I had escaped a situation of complete humiliation and learned a lot. Perceptive, constructive, kind people like Sara could find ways to help without making me feel completely helpless. I could survive very difficult situations and could even find humor in seemingly total disasters. These were critical lessons that would prove to make it much easier to cope with my situation and my challenges.

I got the severed bolt fixed and was back to normal the next day. I even had more dates with Sara, but I was still way behind my peers in the dating category, and that did not change until I got to college.

Everyone, it seemed, started to see the humor in my life with Herbie. As we drove from Detroit to the coast of Maine for our annual two-week family vacation that summer, some funny things happened. For long drives, I didn't wear my leg. On the way to

Maine, driving in our Ford LTD station wagon, we displayed Herbie out one of the back, side windows and watched the faces of drivers that passed us on that side. The classic double take was quite common and hilarious to us on long tedious drives. It really did look like a body was lying there.

We stopped somewhere in Quebec and stayed in a hotel. Some hotels were not too happy about Lobo staying with us. Refusing to have him spend the night in the car, I donned my sunglasses, put white tape on my cane, and tried to get Lobo to act like a disciplined seeing-eye dog. If I went pretty fast (for a blind man) past the registration desk, I could get away with it. Of course, Lobo knew nothing about acting like a seeing-eye dog, and so no one paying attention would have been fooled for a second. But I got away with it anyway. Lobo was always well-behaved and never barked in the room, so all I had to do was get us past the desk and we were home free.

Greenings Island in Maine was a place of safe exploration into challenging new things I could accomplish. It was a place to strengthen my spirit, my confidence, and my body—especially my arms. The normal mode of transport the one mile from Southwest Harbor to the island was a lobster boat converted into a ferry. The ferry kept to a rigid schedule that did not always suit everyone's needs. So, using one of the islands' several large, sturdy rowboats, I became the alternative off-schedule taxi service, rowing back and forth to town two or three times a day.

To get even more rowing in, I created an event of rowing around Greenings Island. It was an event no one else could do—not even my older brother or my dad—because they had not been working as hard on their arms. Suddenly there was something I was able to do that others would not or could not do. This was a wonderful and startling discovery: it wasn't always going to be about me trying to match what "normal" people could do. I could find things where I could surpass others. This is a dramatic turning point for people with a disability or a disadvantage: when they realize they can be not just good "considering," not even just "good period," but actually better than the average "able-bodied" or "able-minded" person.

Arm strength was a natural offshoot of my body's adaptation to the loss of a limb. Crutch walking and rowing were adding strength and tone to already reasonably strong arms. But it was leg strength that I needed to build up more than anything else. I had skied just three months post-amputation on a tiny bump of a hill in southern Michigan. Although that local resort could hardly be called a "ski area," the experience was enough to highlight the importance of leg strength and endurance. After skiing a few runs, I would get a lactic acid burning sensation in my leg that was so severe I had to sit down. After resting, I would do it again. And again and again. Once past the leg burning sensation, the next stage was uncontrollable shaking, after which came involuntary total collapse. It happened fast. One minute I'd be skiing along upright, the next minute my leg would be shaking, and—boom—I was on the ground. That led to the final stage of complete exhaustion: major cramps. Rock-hard, painful, long-lasting cramps. Going through that a few times provided all the motivation I needed to get my leg a heck of a lot stronger.

It is hard for two-legged people to fully appreciate what it's like to ski, bike, hike, or do any activity for a long time on one leg. Or, for that matter, with any kind of physical disability that removes a part of the body from productive output. A two-legged person naturally shifts weight back and forth between their two legs. That way, one is usually resting. Even standing at a party or in line at a supermarket checkout, two-leggers constantly shift weight from one leg to another so they can last longer. While they eventually will get tired, it's nothing compared to what happens to someone standing on one leg, unable to shift weight. That is the story for amputees. A modified story with the same theme applies to anyone with a limb loss, deformity, or impairment.

During my senior year of high school, Judy Bjorndal, a medical student, lived with us. She was a student at Wayne State, where my parents taught, and they decided to host her and have her live with us. She was a complete jock. Tennis mostly. She was tall, thin, and very nice, but had a toughness to her personality that manifested itself as not giving other people too much sympathy in which to wallow. Her expectations of people were quite high. I was no exception. Her attitude toward my situation rubbed off on many people around me. She was very good for me.

Judy's approach to getting my leg in tip-top shape exemplified her attitude. She became my personal trainer, right there in our house. She devised leg-strengthening activities that were grueling for two-leggers, and that much more so for me, but they were not out of reach. She had me work toward leg strength that exceeded a goal to which most two-leggers would aspire. Her approach was instrumental in my development of the right mindset for physical activities. Someone like Judy is what anyone with a disability needs on his or her support team.

Judy's plan started with lots of rope jumping combined with hopping up and down stairs. A side benefit was great one-legged balance. I worked out with her in the evenings. She pushed and pushed me. I jumped rope for a count of one hundred and then rested. Then I hopped down and up the stairs to the basement. Next, I did phantom chair sits against the wall on the one leg until it shook and collapsed. Finally, I went back to the jump rope and repeated the entire regimen three times.

My leg gained four inches in circumference. I was able to jump rope for five minutes without stopping. I learned jump rope tricks I had never perfected on two legs, like crossover jumping. In crossover jumping, the arms cross over each other while the rope is overhead, and then when the rope comes back around underfoot, the jumper's arms are fully crossed across their chest. The next cycle they come uncrossed and so on each time around. When done well, it becomes a smooth circular motion with the hands. I eventually learned to do crossovers where my hands stayed crossed. I even learned to do double jumps with my hands crossed over. I did crossovers jumping backwards and even double jumps backwards crossed over. Even the most proficient rope jumpers find this challenging to do on two legs, much less balancing on one.

Jumping rope was the way my leg ultimately got the majority of its strength and endurance that enabled me to excel in sports like skiing and biking. Then, doing each of these sports took that leg strength and endurance to the next level. Once muscles are significantly developed, it is much easier to maintain that level. From that point in time, my leg has never gotten smaller again. It goes through cycles of being in more or less good shape for specific sports, which is mostly a question of endurance and not strength.

I was making discoveries at a rapid pace. I figured out how to play softball respectably. The best position for me was pitcher.

I needed to have a pinch runner when I batted, but I could hold my own. I played at every picnic I attended. Years later it was the centerpiece activity at my wedding, as soon as the ceremony was over and we could get out of our wedding clothes.

On crutches, I had no disadvantage in hiking relative to two-leggers other than a practical distance limit. On each trip to Maine, we picked a couple mountains on the big island of Mt. Desert to hike during the week. I made a few adaptations to avoid skin blisters and abrasions on these long, tough, steep hikes. One was to wear a large piece of mole foam under my armpit where the crutch pads rubbed. If I didn't, the skin would rub off and bleed. I also learned to wear tight sports tape—not gloves—on my hands so no rubbing would occur to create blisters. With these two adaptations, I could hike as long as my arm endurance lasted. That limit turned out to be ten to twelve miles, but six was most comfortable. Since most hikers average about two miles per hour, three-hour hikes are about all most people like to do in one stretch anyway.

With more than the usual late-teenager feeling of immortality, my sense of invincibility was growing, and with it I was beginning to lose my sense of fear. This was most true with athletic activities. Sailing is a good example. I did some crazy sailing stunts when we were vacationing on Greenings Island, sailing the ocean waters out of Southwest Harbor. We had a little Sunfish sailboat. We also had access to a nice wooden gaff rig boat called the White Cap. I always liked how close to the edge of disaster you were in a small boat like the Sunfish. Lose your concentration in a Sunfish and you will capsize in Maine's extremely cold water. You don't just set the sail, pick a course, and steer like in a larger boat. You constantly have to watch the wind and your sail, adjusting the main sheet and the tiller to keep right on the edge between spilling wind out of the sail and collecting too much wind, which results in tipping you over.

I spent a lot of time in that boat, frequently taking Lobo with me. He sat very still and calm in the cockpit. Sometimes he would see a seal surface near us and get excited and bark. The seals sometimes even barked back.

I liked to push the envelope and see how far out toward open water I could go. With many islands off Mt. Desert Island providing protection, there was little open water swell. But if I went out far enough—perhaps ten miles—I started to feel the big swells. I had no instruments, no equipment of any kind, and, I am afraid, no brains. Storms can and did come up fast. There were times when the strong gale force winds came roaring in and blew the water flat and black. When that happened, the wind usually came onshore, so I could set the sail out perpendicular to the side of the boat—a tack called "running free"—to get back home. The original design of the Sunfish was based on a surfboard. A strong wind from behind makes the hull plane on the surface of the water like surfing. Any more wind, however, and the boat can tumble head over heels. Had that happened in a black wind, I would have been a goner.

I had many close calls doing extreme sailing, but my mortality was no longer something that entered my mind, so I kept doing things that went right up to and then just over the edge. The more accomplished I felt in not just recovering from an amputation and beating cancer, but also routinely doing things that two-legged people couldn't or wouldn't do, the more I ignored worrying about risk, danger, or dying. Risk taking became an addiction.

The winter of 1975 was time to reap the benefits (I hoped) of all the rope jumping and leg strength training. I headed to Mt. Tremblant in Quebec for the family ski vacation—a big step up from the local ski hill in Michigan. I now had outriggers, which are Canadian or forearm crutches with small ski tips where normally there would be crutch tips. I had to learn how to use the outriggers correctly. Riding the T-bar was a big challenge; I needed a free hand to catch and hold the bar, but I also needed an outrigger riding on the snow to keep balanced on the speedy ride up the mountain. Once skiing down I was determined to make my left and right turns symmetrical; the left turns were still clumsy compared to the right. Even with the outriggers and my increased leg strength, much to my disappointment my leg still became exhausted and cramped up by the middle of the afternoon. I had a lot to work on, but overall it was a trip full of experimentation, new discoveries, and exciting progress. People I skied past stared, but for once I found I didn't mind that so much.

Frequently someone would say, "I wonder if you can do X." Or worse, they would say, "I bet you can't do Y." That pretty much sealed my fate that I would spend a lot of time getting good at Y. I was like that kid everyone knew in elementary school who would do dumb things on a dare because he so wanted to prove himself to everybody. Waterskiing was one of those things. Someone suggested that I would never be a good water skier. I had tried it at various lake retreats over the years prior to the loss of my leg, but we usually had wimpy boats and I never had anyone actually coach me. Focused on this new mission, I made friends with some guys who were good water skiers and whose family had a boat. Most importantly, they were interested (and patient) enough to see if it could be done well by someone on one leg.

Most beginners who want to slalom ski will start with two skis and drop one once they are up and steady. Getting up on two skis is much easier for the skier and it requires less effort from the boat as well. Even a strong slalom skier getting up on one ski can use the free leg to help get himself out of the water. In contrast, I am a big dead weight on the boat because my one and only foot is locked into the ski, and I have no spare leg to kick and help get to the surface. Boat drivers had to understand this and be very patient. To them it looked like I couldn't possibly come up because I would submarine for such a long way before suddenly popping up. I have had many drivers kill the motor just as I was about to pop up because they did not think it was working. Getting up on one ski took many tries while I figured out the timing and the balance. It was a good thing my arms were strong from crutch walking because the pull from the boat as I was dragged underwater was intense.

Persistence is the best friend to someone facing a disability. It became a theme for me, and it remains so to this day in whatever I do. In waterskiing, I finally got to the point where I could get up slalom on the first try every time. I modified my ski to have the back boot removed and the front one slipped back a few inches, allowing my one foot to have some leverage over the back of the ski it needed for hard cuts across the wake. Because I lack the back foot that helps make hard turns, my cuts across the wake are not quite as tight as I like, but I get back and forth across the wake pretty quickly and can ski a long time.

An activity to which I did not get back for a while, post amputation, was swimming. I am not sure why, especially given how important it later became. It probably had to do with it being a sport in which I competed well as a sprinter, and sprinters use both legs very aggressively. When I finally got competitive again, it was only after I had converted myself from a sprinter into a long-distance swimmer. In long-distance swimming, the main job of the legs is to keep the whole body level and on the water's surface. They do little in the way of propulsion. My adaptation was to wear a flipper and to kick in a crisscross pattern that allowed the one leg to keep my lower body on the surface while using a kicking pattern that kept me going in a straight line without fishtailing.

As I became more comfortable walking with the artificial leg, and more comfortable with my relationships with other people, I found interesting (and sometimes funny) ways to use my situation to make a point. At the end of high school, I had a summer job building artificial trees at Frank's Nursery in Detroit. My coworker, Dave, and I were tasked with creating a realistic tree from an assortment of parts: a plastic tree made in Taiwan wrapped up tight in shrink-wrap, a real redwood pot, a tree holder to place inside the pot, foam to fill space inside the pot, and some organic moss to cover all the fake bits. When taken out of their tight, plastic sleeves, the tree branches had to be pulled down into a realistic tree shape. This job was filled with opportunities for creativity. We assemblers had to be real artistes to create a live-looking tree—one that was worthy of a gas station or cheap hotel's lobby. Dave was what we called "a stoner." He liked to come to work stoned, get stoned at lunch, and leave work stoned. He also liked to crawl into the back of the warehouse and take naps while I worked and kept a watchful eye out for our boss, Gordy. Gordy made that easy because he always came into our warehouse building driving a forklift, which we could hear from a mile away. I quickly became a little resentful of Dave and his laziness.

One step in the tree construction process was to create a holder for the trunk of the plastic tree that would firmly sit in the bottom of the redwood tub. To do this, we took cardboard tubes and fired a bunch of staples through the side of the cardboard cylinder toward its center at an angle; when we pushed the tree trunk down into the tube, all of the angled staples grabbed hold so that the trunk could not be pulled back out of the tube. Then all we had to do was make sure the tube itself stayed firmly planted on the bottom of the wooden tub. We used our air-powered staple gun again to accomplish this, stapling through from the outside bottom of the tub and up into the cardboard tube. Voila, an artificial tree root system.

One day I noticed stoner Dave just staring off into space. I was sitting in front of the jig we used to hold a trunk-stabilizing tube, onto which we placed an upside-down wooden pot for stapling. I was doing ten pots to every one of Dave's. I got frustrated, I got mad, and I wanted to make a point. I placed a cardboard tube on the jig, put a redwood pot upside down on top of it, got my high-powered staple gun, spun the tub and tube assembly, and rat-a-tat-a-tat, I put a nice ring of staples through the tub as it revolved around in a complete circle. Then I just kept going. I let the staple gun run right up my wooden leg from my knee to my hip. Dave gasped and literally fell over backwards. In seconds he was up and running—quite nimble and quick for someone so stoned—to get Gordy and first aid help, assuming my leg would be gushing blood any second.

When I heard the forklift announcing Gordy's arrival from the building two hundred feet away, I was using a screwdriver to pry the staples out of my wooden leg. I had some holes in my blue jeans and my balsa wood leg, but otherwise no harm was done. Except, perhaps, to Dave's psyche.

We loved to pile empty boxes as we unloaded each shipment of plastic trees. We were supposed to smash the boxes as we unloaded them, but rules be damned. Instead we created a huge pile twenty feet across and eight feet high. We would climb up one wall to the crossbeam and, hanging from the beam with our feet about six feet from the top of the pile, inch our way out until we were directly over the boxes. Then we'd drop into the pile, letting the boxes break an otherwise fourteen-foot drop onto concrete. And my poor prosthetics team wondered why I seemed to be so much harder on my leg than any of their other patients.

Fire extinguisher wars were our other favorite pastime. The fire extinguishers were the kind that were filled with water and pressurized, so it was easy to recharge them after use and there was no mess to clean up. Whenever Gordy was nowhere to be found and we needed a break from the artificial tree production line, Dave or I would grab the nearest extinguisher and start blasting the other. In no time, one of us would be soaked. I am sure all that water in the knee mechanism was not ideal for my leg, but at the time I didn't care much about that. What I did care about was that I could hold my own, do anything the other guy was doing, and have a lot of fun after the lonely years of high school.

By the time I reached graduation, I was perhaps more ready to be done with high school than any other schoolmate with the worst case of senioritis. It was a time and a set of experiences I wanted to put behind me. I had not done well with friends who had treated me as if I were a leper. There had been very little dating. Social interactions with my age group had been minimal. The good things had been limited to academics, a little athletics, my escape into music, and summer activities like camp and family vacations.

I was now down to using just a cane with Herbie. I had gotten strong, taken up many of the sports I had loved before, and started doing some new things that allowed me to participate with other active people. My confidence was growing. Walking on my prosthesis was—and still is—the most nerve-racking thing I had to do. In fact, my biggest fear on graduation day was that I would walk across that stage to pick up my diploma and wipe out, taking the principal down with me. In the end, I celebrated a successful walk across the stage even more than I celebrated earning my high school diploma.

High school and all it entailed lingered as a difficult and mostly negative experience for me. I needed the clean slate of going away to college and leaving all that was high school behind. I chose Kalamazoo College in the western part of Michigan. My older brother attended there too, but my decision to apply had nothing to do with him. I wanted a school that was smaller than my high school and far enough away that I would not feel pressured to come home too often, yet I still wanted it to be within a reasonable driving distance. I applied for early decision to Kalamazoo; I was not the slightest bit interested in any other school.

Kalamazoo followed the quarter system of ten-week terms. During the fall quarter of my freshman year, I went on a wild burst of speed dating. I had figured out the prosthesis to a certain extent, and I had gained some confidence. It felt like the right time to try to catch up socially. With $1,000 to my name from being an artificial tree artiste, I proceeded to go on forty dates in ten weeks. I went out every Thursday, Friday, Saturday, and Sunday night—never with the same girl twice. I was absolutely fearless (or shameless) about asking girls out on dates. I went up to complete strangers in the cafeteria or walked across the quad to ask a name and for a date. Many said yes, but I didn't mind if they said no. I was driven. Little did they know they were part of a major transformation I was going through.

I was determined to learn to dance with my prosthesis. That was no mean feat on a wooden leg in those days. Now the computerized prostheses make dancing relatively safe, but back then the legs were strictly designed for straight ahead walking on level ground and not the back and forth gyrations of rock and roll dancing. It was my new "mission impossible." I may have been determined, but I was not yet facile enough with the leg to dance and not fall. So I fell. A lot. The poor girls had no idea what was about to happen when they agreed to a date with me. On the dance floor, my focus and determination trumped embarrassment. Sometimes we'd be the only ones out on the dance floor, which normally is an intimidating prospect, but with me falling it must have been totally humiliating—for her. I, on the other hand, was in some parallel universe where I suddenly did not care. We'd dance for a while and then, crash, I'd suddenly find myself on the floor. I was constantly shocked and amazed at how fast gravity worked. My dates looked alternately embarrassed, worried, shocked, and sympathetic. They looked around to see how many people were staring at us, then they assumed I wanted to stop and go sit down. I got up and apologized, but kept going. Sometimes I wouldn't even tell my dates I had an artificial leg. They probably figured I had a bad knee, unless the word was out and everyone already knew why I limped. No wonder I had no second dates. I wasn't particularly interested in second dates, although if I ever wanted to lose my virginity before I turned twenty (which I hoped for but wouldn't achieve), I would have to get off the first date kick. Still, my method was proving something very important to me about normalcy, acceptance, and courage—all of which I felt I badly needed in order to fully recover.

There was an aspect of catching up on a lot of lost time with this frenzy. I was dating, but none of this turned into even a hint of a relationship. There was barely even any kissing. It was almost like an event in which I just had to participate. After ten weeks of four dates a week, with me always paying even in an age of Dutch dates, I had run through my $1,000. Also, for the first time ever, I was not getting good grades.

I was given an exemption to the rule that freshman couldn't have cars on campus. Plus, I got great parking spots thanks to the handicapped placard I had finally gotten. At first I wanted nothing to do with a handicapped placard because I hated the word "handi-capped" and didn't want to be associated with people "like that." I eventually changed my tune because I began to feel like I had earned that placard and the convenience it provided. Ironically, I needed the placard most when I was wearing my leg because it was long-distance walks with the prosthesis that were hardest. When I first went in to apply for it, I did not have to have a doctor's letter because the official rule stated that if my condition was "completely obvious to a lay person," no doctor's approval was needed. When I went to the desk at the DMV office and handed the lady my form with the "it's obvious" checkbox checked, she stood up and looked over the desk and down at my legs to see just how obvious this was. I never wore shorts so, not seeing anything amiss, she turned me down. "You can't do that. I'm wearing a prosthesis," I said. "Oh, in that case let me come around and see it," she replied. So right there in the crowded DMV office, there she was, down on her knees, feeling up my leg. First she felt the wooden leg, and then she moved left and started to feel up my real leg. I quickly explained that I had the problem only on one side and the left side was quite real, thank you. I got the placard and have had one ever since. I get occasional looks from people who see me driving a car with a placard and assume from my face and upper body that I must be a scam artist parking in those spots. But when I get out with crutches, their expressions change quickly. It's especially disconcerting for passersby when I have two kayaks on top of my car, two bikes on the back, and still park in a handicapped spot.

Having the car, having it right there in front of the dorm, and having access to the best parking places at bars, movies, and restaurants resulted in a lot more friends than I realized I had. My age group slipped through a brief period when Michigan had changed the legal drinking age from twenty-one to eighteen, and it only changed back after I was twenty-one. We were part of a very lucky partial generation that was allowed to drink when we were eighteen. We took advantage of it and went to bars a lot.

A very distinct difference from high school was that in college I was forming lasting friendships that would survive even bigger challenges than the loss of my leg. Dave Francis, whom I never roomed with, became my best friend during college. We were pretty sure that rooming together would have destroyed our friendship. Dave was smart and eventually earned his PhD in clinical psychology. Later he would run the psychology department at the University of Houston. He was also very good at pool. A game room under the dining hall had two pool tables. Dave and I were both good students, and we both had mostly morning classes, so we tried to get most of our studying done before dinner. We also always got to dinner when the doors opened at 4:30 sharp. Dinner was the best social time of the day, and Dave and I held court at a large round table through at least three seatings of other students rolling through dinner. We kept drinking coffee as shift after shift of our friends flowed through to eat their dinner, visit for a while, and go off to study while we got ready to entertain the next group.

After three or four shifts, we moved downstairs to the pool tables. A solid two hours of pool and it was time for a little studying, but not too much, followed by a visit to the snack bar or a pizza and beer in my room with some great music. You can be sure spending two hours a day playing pool results in an improved game. Dave was better than me, but I was still good enough. We plied our trade occasionally in Kalamazoo's local pool and drinking establishments. Dave was good at miscuing when we first got up to the table, so invariably someone, thinking they had some poor local college weenies at their mercy, challenged us to a game. Losers bought beer. We almost never had to pay for our beer. But more than once we got chased out for scamming people. At times the chasing was not so gentle, and I would feel the rush of wind from a cue stick as it swiped close to the back of my head.

I bounced around several majors at college: physics, history, and finally math. Math had been the best subject for me in high school. I was inspired in high school by my calculus teacher, Mr. Temple, and in college by Dr. Thomas Jefferson Smith who made math fun and challenging. These two teachers were directly responsible for my love of math and for me eventually getting a PhD in computer science.

On the quarter system, most students just attended three out of four quarters and took the first summer off. But I went eight quarters straight without taking off a single quarter. I rarely went home. Home had some difficult associations for me in spite of the great support my parents had provided me in the worst of times. When I needed a break, I was more likely to go to Naperville, Illinois, where my aunt kept a very inviting place for me to relax. I was still putting distance between myself and high school, parents, events, and places that were wrapped up in the loss of my leg.

Barney McKee, my brother's roommate, and I became very good friends. After my brother got married at the end of my freshman year, Barney and I decided to drive to Maine and hang out on Greenings Island where my family had gone for so many years. Barney and I had a meticulously planned college student getaway. He drove a yellow pickup truck with huge fire decals down its sides. It was a standard transmission, so on the surface it seemed like something a one-legger couldn't drive. But with twenty-two hours one way from Detroit to Mt. Desert Island, Maine, it was too much for Barney to drive himself. So we figured out a way for me to drive a standard transmission with some maneuvers that would make even James Bond proud.

The hard part with a manual transmission is starting from a dead stop in first gear. That is the only time you need both feet at the same time for the clutch and accelerator. Once the car is moving, the driver can easily shift up through the gears without having to "feather" the accelerator. So, with a full tank of gas, Barney got us going on the freeway, and then we traded places while the truck was moving at full speed in high gear. It worked like a charm. I drove for hours while he got a rest, and I never needed to use both feet at the same time.

Once we got there, we craved lobsters, as does everyone when they are in Maine in the summer. The problem was that we were poor college students who could in no way afford lobster. We decided not to let that stop us. Going out in a motorboat and poaching lobsters from traps would be illegal, immoral, and suicidal. So we came up with a different plan that was illegal, immoral, and suicidal, not to mention weird. We went out in the sailboat at night, without any lights whatsoever. I sailed and looked for running lights on potential collision targets, while Barney pulled up a lobster trap with his bare hands and checked out its contents. Real lobster fisherman, besides never fishing at night without lights and never in a sailboat, also never pull up their traps by hand. They use power winches instead. We each wanted two two-pound lobsters, so anything small we found we just threw back. It took maybe ten trap pulls to find what we wanted, making our exposure out on the water with no running lights longer and more dangerous, not to mention that Barney's hands were sore and bleeding from pulling up the heavy lines. We feared that if a lobsterman caught us poaching his traps, he would not hesitate to shoot us, tie cement to our feet, and drop us overboard. This was his livelihood, and there would be no waiting for the slow wheels of justice for these hardscrabble Mainers. Nobody ever caught us and we succeeded in getting four two-pounders, just as we had hoped.

The next morning we planned a feast out at the tip of the island where we could look out toward open ocean while we cooked and ate. We cooked the lobsters in seaweed on the rocks and ate them with cornbread and salad. It was magnificent, made even more so by the dangerous acquisition of the food. Never had lobster tasted so good. Four pounds of lobster is quite a bit, even for big, strong, growing college boys. We were in college student heaven.

We rowed. We hiked. We sailed. Friends like Barney, who didn't make a special deal about my disability, in some ways made the disability disappear. Barney integrated smoothly into his thinking and planning what I could do and what I could not do. I sometimes wore my prosthesis and sometimes left it off, depending on the activity we were doing. I was not yet comfortable being seen on crutches in public settings like stores or restaurants, but on the island, while sailing and especially on the hiking trail, I was fine with it. While on crutches there were times when carrying something that could easily spill was best done by the person with two legs. People close to me figured that out without making me feel crippled when they carried it for me. And when I was wearing my leg, those same people knew not to suggest we walk six blocks to a movie or a store. There is a real knack to smoothly integrating these behaviors, especially when the disabled person's situation is so dynamic as mine was.

THREE

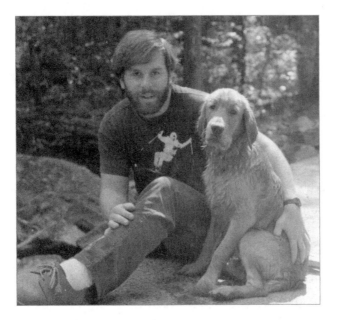

ZERO CHANCE OF SURVIVAL

A cancer is not only a physical disease, it is a state of mind.

— Michael M. Baden, physician, author

The more serious the illness, the more important it is for you to fight back, mobilizing all your resources—spiritual, emotional, intellectual, physical.

— Norman Cousins, essayist

This is like déjà vu all over again.

— Yogi Berra, baseball player and manager

During my sophomore year of college, disaster struck while I was home for the holidays. I needed to get my wisdom teeth out during Christmas break. I arranged to get only one side—top and bottom—done to start with; I had seen people in total misery when they had all their wisdom teeth extracted at once. I was on vacation, after all, and wanted to be able to chew real food after the procedure, albeit only on one side of my mouth. While I was at the hospital, I had my routine blood test and chest X-ray that I had been getting every six months since the cancer's onset three years previously. I went for these checkups because I had to, but, like any teenager who feels at best immortal and at worst blissfully ignorant, I did not feel the slightest risk of a recurrence. On the day my wisdom teeth were extracted, I went first for the cancer screening tests, and then I went downstairs and was put under general anesthesia for the oral surgery. The oral surgeon knew my father well, as always seemed to be the case in the Detroit medical community.

While I was still in the dentist chair and coming out from under the anesthesia, I had a visitor from the lab upstairs who ominously and dramatically said I was not to leave the hospital. They admitted me into the hospital that afternoon, right from oral surgery, stitches and all. Then came the punch line—sucker punch, really. The cancer had spread to my lung. For three years, these routine tests had been clean. Meanwhile, my adaptations to the disability and confidence had grown steadily. But that confidence, and my world, came crashing down in seconds.

I honestly thought the six-month checkups were silly—overprotectiveness of my parents and doctors—and nothing was ever going to show up. Now something had shown up. They discovered a lung mass on the chest X-ray, and it was an all out emergency to get the metastasized tumor in my lung removed—pronto. Their worst fear—and mine—that the cancer had spread through the bloodstream to a new site, had now come true.

They kept me busy in the hospital room that night, prepping me for the next day's surgery. This included a major amount of shaving, even though at nineteen I had very little chest hair. It reinforced where they were going to cut me open: right across the side of my ribcage. This was in some ways a scarier prospect than even the amputation of my leg. For one thing, it was "closer to home" to where all my vital organs were located. For another, I found frightening the prospect of them cutting into my lungs when breathing is such a vital second-by-second bodily function. Difficulty catching a breath is one of the most instinctive human fears. I was petrified, yet beyond crying. I was numb with fear. It wasn't just fear of the surgery the next day. This cancer was not letting me go. Everything I felt three years before came back with a vengeance. All the confidence I had started to regain was instantly wiped out. Sleep was not restful; it was pure psychic exhaustion.

Early the next morning I was scheduled for a procedure called a "thoracotomy" to remove two-fifths—or the lower lobe—of my left lung. Humans have a big and a medium lobe on the left side (to leave room for one's heart) and three small ones on the right side. I was having the largest one removed, so it amounted to losing about two-fifths of my total lung capacity.

Here I was again in a hospital room waking up to a flurry of pre-surgery activity. It was déjà vu, except for the fact that déjà vu is supposed to be an illusion and this was very real. I had been here just three years ago. *What would happen in another three years? What body part would be next? Would I even be around in three years? In three months?* These were sentiments I had not had with the first bout of cancer.

This time my parents were more obviously scared. They tried to appear strong to help bolster me, but their efforts were futile. They were devastated and seemed without hope. Once again, the nurses got me groggy and wheeled me down to the operating room. This time I decided to be a wise guy and count forward. Strangely it helped to pretend I was somehow in control and an old hand at this surgery stuff.

They performed the surgery from my back and side so they didn't have to crack as many ribs. Still, crawling inside my chest cavity did a lot of collateral damage, all of which turned into pain once I was awake. It also created quite a scar—about fifteen inches long—that follows the line of my shoulder blade around to my left side. They cut through muscles, so recovery was difficult. It affected my breathing, of course, but it also affected any movement that involved my core or my left arm. Sneezing or coughing was excruciating. The surgery also cut many nerves, so a lot of skin near the scar no longer has any sensation.

This time I was much more aware of my surroundings even in the recovery room. I came up fighting immediately. Right away they told me I had to pee and said if I could not they would have to put in a catheter. It all sounded too familiar. I hated those things, but the body just does not work very well after a long bout with anesthesia. I kept standing up to try to pee and just couldn't. They threatened and I tried again. They went to get the catheter equipment and I finally managed to do it myself. I was going to fight back as hard and as fast as I could against anyone or anything that got in the way of my getting strong and healthy again. I was going to fight to the death if necessary.

They told me my stay in the hospital would be quite lengthy because I had chest tubes through my side to drain where the lung had been. The entry sites of those tubes to this day look like bullet hole scars. They said three weeks in the hospital. I said one. It would be a battle to see who was right.

They said it would be hard to raise my left arm over my head, as it would take weeks to repair and build back the cut muscles to perform that motion. I said, "You mean like this?" and raised my arm over my head in spite of excruciating pain. Their jaws dropped: I wasn't supposed to be able to do that for weeks.

Around others, I was tough and determined. But alone, I was the most depressed I had ever been in my short life. I couldn't stop thinking of what was now floating around in my bloodstream. Where would this nasty stuff land next, and what would have to be cut out of me then? Along with the classic "Why me?" question, I was just plain scared. I even started having thoughts that maybe something I had thought or done had promoted the growth of these cells, and I needed to control my thoughts much better to keep this from happening again. However, my depression was about to get much deeper, as what I was thinking was not nearly as bad as what they would tell me next.

Zero chance of survival. That is what I faced. At least, that is what I heard when my doctor said that no one who had had a metastasized osteosarcoma tumor in the lung had survived. In fact, he told me, prior to 1976, no one had ever survived when osteosarcoma metastasized anywhere. They held out one faint glimmer of hope. A new treatment was available that had been in clinical research trials when I lost my leg three years earlier: chemotherapy. I had heard about chemotherapy, and I had certainly heard about radiation therapy. They described these chemotherapy drugs as radiomimetic because they mimic radiation. I would start on the drugs as soon as I recovered enough from the surgery.

I was in Harper Hospital in Detroit. It was a brand new hospital next door to Grace Hospital, where my leg had been amputated. I got a private room at my father's insistence; he was the vice chairman of the department of surgery, and he got what he wanted. I received many visitors, but again no friends my age came to see me. It was easy for my parents to visit because they worked right there. Some of the surgery residents who worked with my dad became friendly with me. My favorite pastime in the hospital was *Mille Bornes*—the French car racing card game. The nurses were nice. Especially nice were the pink-uniformed student nurses. They had to wash me in the bed because I was not very mobile due to the chest tubes connected to the lung suction machine. Breathing was hard, and every breath hurt. Every so often, especially because of some fluid buildup, my body really wanted to take a deep breath that would push air down into the furthest recesses of the lungs. But doing so just hurt too much, so it was a battle between two competing parts of my brain.

I still hated the hospital, and especially hospital food, particularly since I could chew only on one side of my mouth because of the removal of my wisdom teeth. One of the residents took pity on me and asked what I wanted to eat most of all. I told him the truth: I wanted a Whopper and a beer. He got them for me. A fast food hamburger—slightly cold—and a beer—slightly warm—never tasted so good. Luckily no one ever found out so he didn't get into any trouble.

Before I went home, I had to bear one more ignominious assault. I still needed the stitches removed from the oral surgery that had extracted my wisdom teeth. While still in the hospital bed recovering from open chest surgery, I had the dozen stitches behind my molars removed. I still needed to have the wisdom teeth on the other side removed at some time in the future, but that was the least of my worries right then.

Even though (because I was maniacal about it) I got to go home after only a week, I had still missed three weeks of college. And with short ten-week quarters, there was no way to catch up, so that quarter was a lost cause . . . almost.

As a math major, I had a certain set of required courses, and the school offered one of those courses only in winter. If I missed that class, I would not graduate on time. The class was Differential Equations with my favorite professor, Thomas Jefferson Smith. It was T.J. Smith to the rescue again. I took his class from my hospital bed and then from home. This was before email, and T.J. didn't use handouts, he just lectured straight from the chalkboard. So T.J. transcribed his notes onto yellow legal pads and sent them to me by mail. To T.J., this was just what one did under the circumstances. To me, and everyone who observed him, he went way beyond the call of duty and was a credit to the college. I had only the textbook and his notes to get through this class. It is arguably the hardest required class a math major must take. It's a good thing my profession never depended heavily on differential equations or I would have been in trouble. While I passed the course, it was by far the weakest of my math performances during college.

My parents knew from my previous recovery that what I needed most—other than going back to sitting in my big comfortable brown chair playing card games—was something to keep my hands occupied and my brain focused. I needed that critically important cognitive busy signal to help manage my pain. The physical pain was bad, but still it was nothing like the debilitating phantom pain I had for weeks and weeks the last time. What was worse this time was the depression and fear—the psychological pain. My parents had always wanted a color TV, so they bought a gigantic Heathkit color TV that I proceeded to build for them from my new quarters in the palatial basement bedroom that had previously been Michael's. This huge project took four or more hours daily over the remainder of that quarter. It was intensive therapy to help with my recovery. I was good at soldering, but not perfect, and I didn't get the TV put together one hundred percent correctly. Whatever I did wrong left it with a bit of a purple hue to the picture; but it was our first color TV, so everyone was happy about it regardless.

As I started to recover, I needed to find something more to do with my idle time. The Differential Equations class and the color TV kit did not fill my time or take all my energy once I started to bounce back. Just sitting around thinking about what would have to be cut out of my body next, or worse, about my zero chance of survival, was certainly not good either. My dad pulled some strings and got me a job in the vascular surgery lab in his hospital—the same hospital in which I had just been a patient. Carole worked in this lab. At the very nadir of my life, when I felt like there was no future, I was meeting the future love of my life.

Several of my math assignments over the previous few quarters had just begun to use computers. Kalamazoo had access to the time-sharing system across the railroad tracks at Western Michigan University. Our interface to this large DEC computer was an old clunky Teletype machine with round keys that one had to slam hard in order to produce input. In retrospect, these were very simple assignments. While it was very early for computers, I found computer programming exciting and alluring. The job I got in the lab was hanging out in the back room as the geek who programmed the Hewlett-Packard tabletop plotter that masqueraded as a computer. The programming language, a form of Basic, was simple and easy to learn. They had a specific program they needed written, and so I got busy trying to create it for them. My boss was Rodger Higgins, a PhD in Biomedical Engineering from England. He was a fun, dynamic, high energy, optimistic person, who, along with his wife Linda, was very cosmopolitan. They were both a positive influence on me.

The women in the lab, Carole and Nellie, were both married and a little older than me. They were friendly, but I was the infamous son of the vice chairman I.K.—as my father was known around the hospital by his first two initials—who got the job just because of strings being pulled. Like most of the people I met in the medical center, they were a bit afraid of him. He was gruff to staff and medical students, and very demanding of residents who faltered in any way—a crooked tie, for example—even if the resident had been awake for thirty-six hours straight.

Everyone in the lab knew about my cancer, and they knew much more about medicine than I did, so they knew how bad my prognosis was. That led to some unwelcome sympathy and elicited a reaction in me that seemed grumpy, unfriendly, or aloof to them. Computers were rare and someone who even pretended to know something about them was rarer. The combination made me some kind of a strange wizard suitable only for the back room while they tended to the real business of the lab and the patients with their vascular ailments.

I did not acknowledge the death threat overtly. Perhaps the inherent feeling of immortality characteristic of a nineteen-year-old was still acting like a heat shield against entering the atmosphere of normal mortality as I tried to rejoin the planet of the living. I went day-to-day, still worried most about losing a critical body part every three or so years. I had yet to learn about all the harsh, debilitating effects of chemotherapy. This was going to add to my already overwhelming list of physical and psychological challenges.

A little more than a month after surgery, I had recovered enough to start the chemotherapy treatments. My existing upper left lung lobe was healing and expanding to stretch and fill the void left by the larger lower lobe. The ribs they had broken to gain access to my chest cavity were almost healed. The chest tube holes were starting to heal. The long scar from the top of my shoulder blade down my back and around to my left side was still very sore. The scar needed several more months to heal, but it was urgent to get the chemotherapy started as soon as possible to eradicate any metastasizing cells floating in the bloodstream before they landed and infected another part of my body.

When it was time for my first chemotherapy treatment, I did just what I was told like some kind of zombie robot. A robot that knew enough, however, to be afraid. With no idea what to really expect, I was not well prepared. I shook from fear. The nurses in a calm and extremely understated way said, "This will make you sick, dear." This did not begin to prepare me for the truth of it. I sat in a chair that looked much like the chair in which they do routine blood draws in any doctor's office. Using a big needle, they found some nice large veins in my right arm on the inside of the elbow bend. Once that big needle was dripping a simple saline solution into me, they injected the chemotherapy drug into the drip line. This first day they started me on just one drug called Adriamycin. It is bright red and they warned me that it would make my pee the same color for the rest of the day. My body's reaction to this drug, which is really a strong poison, was quick. Before even leaving the chair, I had vomited my entire stomach contents into a little pan they had given me for that purpose. My body wanted nothing to do with the poison. The heaving even after my stomach was empty was convulsive. My mom drove me home. I felt like I had an incredibly bad hangover. I kept throwing up. The world around me spun as we drove through it. I was miserable.

Lying down once we got home seemed to make the world spin harder and faster. I needed to be propped up. I got only fitful sleep. Now I was dealing with phantom pain, incision pain, nausea, and dizziness, not to mention all the psychic challenges swirling around in my head. The next day, I had to do it all over again, but with different drugs. I got sick much faster because my body was already hip to this trick. The third day I got violently sick before the needle even touched my skin. The fourth day included a tingling of my scalp on the way to the doctor's office—a precursor to getting violently ill. This time I got sick just walking in the door. My veins were traumatized from being stuck multiple times and having caustic drugs pushed through them. They switched arms, using different veins in each arm, and they used veins in my wrists. My arms began to look like a junkie's.

It has been more than thirty years since the chemotherapy drugs were in my system, yet just writing about this experience causes a strong visceral reaction. For many years after the treatments, I could not talk about them without getting nauseous. After the first injection, just arriving in the same office for the next injection caused me to vomit. For years if I saw the same rug pattern somewhere else, I would get sick. I bemoaned my brain's inability to control my physical reactions—something that in normal circumstances I thought I was pretty good at. Everyone experienced with these drugs assured me there was nothing I could do. The power of the brain to protect itself and its body is awesome. The brain realized these drugs were poison and activated a reptilian fight-or-flight instinct. While the nausea and vomiting before injections was indeed psychological, it was based on the violent physical reaction that occurred after each injection.

My regimen was to take four drugs every day for five days and then allow my system to recover over the next three weeks. Bone marrow's production of blood cells shuts down during injections. One of the drugs had a deleterious effect on the heart, so the doctors played a balancing act between injecting enough of the drug to kill the bad cells without damaging the heart. Chemotherapy drugs work by attacking fast-growing cells. That includes, among others, hair cells, bone marrow, and cells that line the intestines. I lost the hair on my head, but not my full beard or any other hair that is slower growing. That first week, huge clumps of hair fell out each night on my pillow. After waking up in a nest of my own hair for three mornings, I said enough is enough and shaved my head. My head already looked like the moth-eaten hide of a stuffed animal, so it didn't seem like I could look much worse being bald.

At first, I was quite self-conscious about my bald head and insisted on getting a wig. Dutifully, my parents took me to a wig store and allowed me to pick out a $400 wig, which was one of the more expensive ones. I wore it, but quickly discovered it was very itchy. When it itched, I scratched by poking a pencil under the wig, which lifted the wig up and shifted it around on my head. That made me look completely ridiculous, so I finally just quit wearing it. Later, back at college and not feeling well most of the time, people said that the big guy with a bald head and a full beard walking with a cane looked meaner than the meanest Marine drill sergeant anyone had ever seen. My friends used that to intimidate incoming freshman from then on, telling them that I was a wounded veteran, straight from the Marines, and they better not mess with me.

For five days this was the drill: get an injection, throw up until there was nothing else to throw up, lie around for the rest of the day and night with the worst hangover feeling anyone has ever had, and then get up in the morning to do it all over again. For five days. It took the three weeks after that for my body to rebuild the cells that were destroyed, including the immune cells.

Spring quarter of my sophomore year, I went back to Kalamazoo. Most of my fellow students were starting to plan their foreign study abroad, to commence the fall quarter of their junior year. Again, as in high school, just as I was establishing strong friendships, I was not able to continue those friendships as I wanted. Cancer had interrupted my relationships again. Due to the chemotherapy, I was not going to be able to join them on foreign study—one of the main attractions that made me choose Kalamazoo in the first place. My doctors didn't want me to continue chemotherapy in Europe. Instead, Kalamazoo invented a customized plan just for me. I was to do the Senior Independent Project as a junior and I would do as a senior what is normally Junior Study Abroad.

Relentlessly, after every three weeks off, it was back to the injections for five more days of vomiting and intense hangovers. No drugs could seem to stop me from throwing up. They tried all the man-made drugs for nausea available, but they were all powerless in the face of this gut-wrenching reaction. People opposed to medical use of marijuana need to experience this level of sickness just once and they will immediately reform their views.

In 1976, there was nowhere in the country, including Michigan, where I could legally use marijuana, even for the most justifiable medical reasons. Fortunately, I had an enlightened physician. He sat me down and stunned me with his question: "Do you know what THC is?"

"Yes," I said.

"Well," he said, "do you know where to get it?"

"Sure."

"Ok. I can't give it to you, but if you can get some, take it in any form before your next injection and see if it makes a difference."

So I tried it and it was truly a miracle. Before and since, I have never liked smoking pot much. This was partly because I did not like to put anything traumatic and smoky into my diminished lungs. However, I was sure going to make an exception if that would keep me from being so sick. I smoked a nice, big, fat joint (yes, I inhaled), feeling very justified doing so, and then drove to the doctor's office. Was driving risky under the influence of a joint? Perhaps, but it was a very short drive on slow city streets, and anticipation of getting violently ill was every bit as much a distracting influence on my driving ability.

I saw the throw-up rug, the throw-up nurses, and the throw-up needle, yet under the influence of the THC I had no reaction. The THC couldn't change the fact that poison was being pumped into my body and that later I would certainly be sick, but it broke my psychological reaction and moderated the later overall reaction as no man-made drug had. It helped me feel like I was back in control.

After the injection, I had about thirty minutes before the hard-core reactions overwhelmed the medicinal effects of the marijuana. I scurried off to see my friends Geoff and Patricia. Geoff had been my brother's roommate along with Barney. He had graduated two years previously, but was back at Kalamazoo because his wife Patricia was finishing her degree. They decided that puking in my dorm room with roommates was not the way to go. Not that me sitting on their couch for three or four hours while watching TV and getting sick was their idea of a good time, but they were very empathetic. They were true friends.

Geoff and I were addicted to reruns of *The Wild Wild West* and watched them every one of the five days I received my injections. He and Patricia would eat while I balanced the throw-up bowl on my lap for quick and easy access whenever a wave of nausea swept over me.

Years later, experts in chemotherapy and cancer treatment told me that I had actually been getting about double the needed dose of those four drugs (Adryamicin, Cytoxan, Vincristine, DTIC). These were the early years of chemo, and they were still experimenting with dosages. They preferred erring on the side of a high dose that attacked the remaining cells in the bloodstream, so long as the side effects of the drugs—especially on the heart—were not worse than having cancer recur.

My treatment continued throughout my spring and summer terms. My Kalamazoo professors bent over backwards to accommodate me. They shifted exams out of those five-day periods as much as possible to fit my chemotherapy schedule. If necessary, they gave me take-home exams or make-up exams. They were incredibly flexible and supportive.

When the fall quarter came, all the other juniors went off to France, Germany, Sweden, England, Japan, and even Africa. I went back to the vascular surgery lab to do my Senior Independent Project as a junior so my chemotherapy could continue. I was back with Nellie and Carole, both of whom were still married. Carole still thought I was a pain, but I was older and seemed less like the punk kid she remembered. I began to notice how incredibly smart and pretty she was. I decided to do whatever was necessary to get her to notice and like me and not just think of me as a privileged kid or a geek hacking away on a computer in the back room. I never in my wildest imaginings could have predicted we would have a future together.

This time I wasn't just programming a silly, glorified HP tabletop calculator. My senior project was to create a structured questionnaire program loosely based on artificial intelligence principles that would help the clinicians diagnose vascular diseases. I used a real programming language called String Oriented Symbolic Language (SNOBOL). To this day, I still consider SNOBOL one of the most fun programming languages to use. I had access to a Wayne State University time-sharing system on which I could write, test, and execute SNOBOL programs.

I was still getting chemo injections for five days every three weeks. During those five days, I didn't accomplish much at the lab. My dad thought it would be nice to let me be at home for injections and decided to volunteer to find my veins himself. Like most surgeons, Dad could cut a patient open and take out an appendix in no time, but he was inexperienced when it came to finding a vein for a chemotherapy injection. "Leave the nurse's job to the nurse," I should have insisted. He painfully missed three or four times on each arm before finally hitting a vein. In honor of his success, he took me out for a steak dinner. We ordered Chateaubriand for two. I was so upset and apologetic a few hours later when that entire beautiful cut of meat came right back up. It seemed like a real waste of delicious meat and money. He was great about it. He said the important thing was how it tasted going down, not whether it stayed down, and certainly not how it tasted coming back up.

In December, after ten months of chemotherapy, they stopped the treatment precipitously because my EKG readings began to show damage to my heart. *Great*, I thought, *something new to worry about for the rest of my life.* All I could do was hope the chemo had enough time to be effective. But with electrocardiogram abnormalities (early indications of possible heart damage) showing up, there was no question the injections had to stop immediately.

Nothing tied me to Detroit or Kalamazoo or anywhere for that matter. I needed to escape. My doctors said I was going to die—not in so many words, but that is what I believed. It was all I could think about. I had not planned this, but now that I was done with the chemo, I wanted to get away. Far away. Finishing college receded to unimportant. I became consumed by a desire to ski. I knew it was going to take me forever to solve my amputee skiing technique issues if I skied only a week or so a year. So I wanted to ski until I could ski no more. I wanted to tackle skiing and get it right. If I could spend an entire season at it, I felt I might be able to get to the point where I was considered a great skier. Period. Not great "considering." Just great.

That December of 1976, I loaded up my green Ford Maverick and, with $1,000 in my pocket and hardly a goodbye to anyone, I started driving west. I believed I could get a job when I got there, but I had nothing lined up. I longed for the life of a ski bum. I had seen such jobs when we went to Alta on a family ski vacation. I didn't actually believe I was going to return. The doctors had just reminded me that they had no idea if chemotherapy worked on this kind of cancer, plus the course was supposed to have run a year and we had to stop it after only ten months. They told me my chances of surviving were slim. I handled all that by wanting to get the hell away and go skiing until I dropped dead.

FOUR

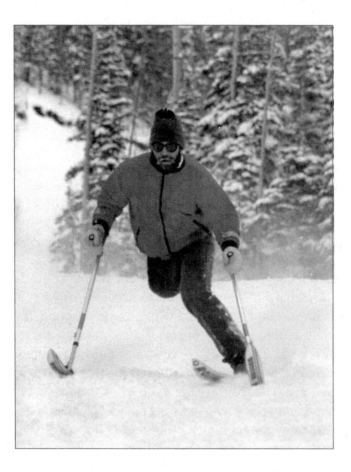

SKI 'TIL I DROP (DEAD)

Live life so completely that when death comes to you like a thief in the night, there will be nothing left for him to steal.

— Anonymous

People have vast potential. Most people can do extraordinary things if they have the confidence or take the risks. Yet most people don't. They treat life as if it goes on forever.

— Philip Adams, broadcaster

saw a romantic appeal in the idea that I would ski until I dropped dead. They had made it clear that I had zero chance of survival based on the old way of dealing—or not dealing—with the cancer once it had spread to the lung. They had high hopes for the chemotherapy, but they did not know for sure it would work. I had gone three years thinking all their tests were just a formality and that nothing bad would happen. Now that something bad had happened, I was no longer the optimist. I wasn't fatalistic either. At nineteen, it's hard to shake the fundamental belief that you are immortal. But if I was going to die, I wanted to accomplish something that was truly important to me first. I wanted to be so good at skiing on one leg that people would just say, "Gosh, he's a great skier," not "Wow, he's good *considering*." I knew it would take many days of skiing, focusing, and working hard to eliminate that word. I needed to improve my balance through the bumps. I needed to take my strength and endurance to an entirely new level. I wanted to be able to ski steep and deep with the best of them. Most of all, I wanted to dramatically refine my skills so my turns were symmetrical, crisp, and fast. In the meantime, I would be doing something I loved, and after the year I had just had, I needed that more than anything.

I never worried what hard, athletic activity at high altitude would mean with only three-fifths normal lung capacity. I had a pulmonary function test just before I left as part of a normal checkup (including those now not so routine chest X-rays and blood tests). When they asked me to breathe in deeply and push as hard as I could on the measuring tube, my competitive juices started flowing. I took a huge breath, steeled myself for the hardest push of my life, and let her rip. I practically turned my lungs inside out. I wanted to break that damn machine and show them. The nurse looked at me as if the reading could not be right. Either that, or I was some kind of freak. She said, "You are at 110 percent of normal capacity." Again, much to my delight, it was not 110 percent considering I only had one lung. It was 110 percent of what someone with two full lungs at my age, height, and weight should be able to do. This gave me some confidence that my lungs could adapt to hard skiing at ten thousand feet.

I cannot say what was going through my parents' heads as I prepared for my departure. I never asked or even consulted with them about leaving. I should have expected a conversation that went something like this:

"I'm going to Alta to be a ski bum."

"Oh, good idea. Do you have a job? Have you saved some money? Where will you stay? Is your car in good shape? When will you go? When will you come home?"

However, we discussed nothing of the kind. Discussing it might have seemed like asking permission, and I was not asking anyone anything. I just went. I was totally self-focused and in self-preservation mode. It was just a few weeks before Christmas. In spite of the fact that Dad was Jewish, we celebrated Christmas and made it a family-focused occasion. But I would not be with them, and never even gave my timing a second thought. They didn't argue or in any way try to dissuade me. They quietly knew they had to stay out of my way. They seemed to know instinctively that I had to go and they had to let me go or risk alienating me. They of all people knew the chemotherapy might not work. They knew they might never see me alive again, yet still they supported what I felt I had to do. Perhaps they realized that if my cancer relapsed, it would happen slowly and they could come get me. Behind my back, and after I was gone, my mother must have been a wreck. I almost never called to give her relief either. She must have worried if I was depressed, had driven carefully, and if I skied carefully (which I didn't). As a parent myself now, I know how completely selfless my parents' support was and how immensely difficult it must have been to give.

On December 6, just days after stopping chemotherapy, I loaded up my beloved green Maverick and started driving. My only travel plan was to drive eight hours per day as if it were a job. I started west on I-94 from Detroit, jumped down onto I-80 at Chicago, and kept driving west until I got to Salt Lake City. I found cheap motels to conserve my money and just kept moving steadily west until I got to Alta, Utah.

I picked Alta because I had been there with my family on ski trips at least twice pre-amputation, and I had loved the powder but found it a challenge. While we were there, I had witnessed a wait staff of very happy ski bums. I had been to lots of other resorts and had never seen the ski bum situation as good as at Alta. These kids had jobs structured so they had lots of time to ski. Other places that had ski bums had them work at more serious all-day jobs and only allowed skiing on days off. I wanted a way to ski each and every day. So Alta it was. But I had not contacted them ahead of time. I had no job waiting. I didn't even check the weather or snow reports. If I had, I would have noticed that this was probably the worst start to a season Alta had had in decades. They were not even open yet and it was mid-December. Many years, they are able to start some high-country skiing around Halloween. By Thanksgiving, there is usually a decent skiing cover of at least three feet. That December, however, they had no snow at all. The hills were brown.

I was going to Alta to be a ski bum and to ski an entire season so I could be a great skier. Period. Little things, like my parents' feelings, lack of snow, no job waiting, or a finite amount of money to spend, were incidental to my goal. It's not as if I was obsessing over the prospect of dying. I really didn't dwell on it. I didn't bemoan my fate, lash out, or become frozen in either fear or self-pity. It moved to the background, but it underlined everything I did. I became even more of a risk-taker. I became much more driven and determined in what I wanted to accomplish. I felt a sense of urgency about everything. "Hurry up and live" could have been my motto. My focus and drive made me seem selfish. Years later, I learned to soften the edges on that as I felt the death sentence lift but I have no doubt it permanently affected my personality and behavior.

I found driving alone for four days, continuously heading west on I-80, a bit scary. However, this kind of scary was actually a nice emotion for me at that point. It felt good to test myself and take on challenges, especially if most people found them intimidating. It's too much of a cliché to say it made me feel alive, but the sentiment "bring it on" was not an exaggeration of my emerging swagger.

Beating challenges made me feel strong; coming out the other side of a challenge made me feel proud, happy, stronger still, and ready to take on more.

I had packed my Maverick with my ski equipment, some food, and all my clothes, but I had left my stereo and hundreds of albums at home. I brought many tapes, but also listened to the radio. Once I was west of Chicago, all the music was country, so then I stuck with cassette tapes.

During the long hours of driving, I always looked for the next milestone to mark my progress. Actually, that's what I did in all aspects of life: I looked forward to the next trip, the next event, the next day, or the next mile marker. I found comfort and optimism in constantly looking forward. It's natural, of course, when you are driving relentlessly west, but it's what I always did anyway. A particularly dramatic milestone was the Continental Divide. I crossed it at night. I thought they could film moon-walking scenes up there if they wanted to. It was dark, cold, and barren, except for the very large hares all over. Lots of them were road kill, but plenty survived the cars as well as the harsh environment. The place gave me a sense of loneliness and isolation that perfectly matched how I felt.

After four days of driving, I arrived at the Goldminer's Daughter Lodge in Alta, right at the base of the mountain. I noticed that the hills were brown, which is highly unusual for December 10, but still I went inside to find the owner. Of all the lodges, Goldminer's Daughter had the best program for ski bums, which I knew from staying at the lodge next door with the family years earlier and talking to the staff there.

I found the owners and asked for a job. Jim and Alfrede laughed with sad smiles and said, "Look outside and see how brown it is out there? Come back when it's white and we'll talk."

Dejectedly, I drove out of Little Cottonwood Canyon and back down to Salt Lake City. I found a place I could rent by the week down there and stayed for a week of perfectly horrendous blue skies. I watched the TV weather, some movies, and an assortment of dumb daytime shows, frequently darting outside to look for a storm coming from the west. Just a single cloud would have been exciting. I was bored to tears. There was not a blemish on the pure blue sky and no signs of anything as far off as the Pacific Ocean on the weather map. After a week, I got worried I would run out of money and my whole plan would crumble. I couldn't face the thought that I might have to give up on this and head back home.

I called home to see if they had any ideas. Mom suggested I drive to L.A. and stay with her brother and his family to save my money. That was just one long day's drive farther west. Heading out across the desert and through Nevada was strange. It seemed I was heading off the end of the world. Vistas were enormous while I, in my little car, seemed so small. I trusted that car to hold up. It had been through a lot already, and it would have to get through a lot more.

I moved in with Aunt Marietta, Uncle Peter, and four cousins: Lisa, Todor, Pico, and Benjamin. I was a pure mooch, just hanging out waiting and waiting for the weather in Utah to break. First thing each morning, I grabbed the newspaper to check out the weather map, looking for just a hint of a storm coming off the ocean. It was eighty degrees in L.A. and all I wanted was snow. For three weeks— through Christmas and then New Year's—I rode it out at my aunt and uncle's place in the hills above Pasadena.

Uncle Peter was a history professor at Cal Tech. Thanks to him I was able to use Cal Tech's outdoor pool, from where I could see the mountains with every stroke. I was used to Christmas in Michigan; it was so strange to be in t-shirts hanging around outside like it was midsummer.

January 5, the exact anniversary of my lung surgery, I spotted just a hint of a storm off the coast on the newspaper weather map. I didn't bother to check if it really was headed for Alta or, heaven forbid, wait to see if it actually dropped any snow there. I just packed up and drove back to Alta the very next day to arrive there on January 6, the day when they did indeed open up for the season because, thankfully, they had gotten over thirty inches from the storm I had spotted. It was the latest opening Alta ever had.

Of course, I had jumped the gun. Alfrede was just getting organized now that the season could finally begin, so she still had no job for me. That was okay with me; I was just glad to be there and for the chance to ski. I said, "I'll stay in your cheapest room until I run out of money or you give me a job, whichever comes first." She gave me a spot in a four-person dorm room that I would share with random hotel guests. I moved in and got ready to ski.

Unlike eastern forest-covered mountains with cut trails, Alta can open only after thirty inches or more of snow has fallen because these ski runs are on exposed rocky slopes, not on trails cut through forests and cleared of all rocks. With huge boulders strewn all over the trails, it takes that much snow to make it even passable on most trails. As it was, there were still a lot of rocks and dirt showing. Still, I didn't care. Nothing was going to deter me, except running out of money and having to give up. I asked Alfrede about the job every day. I have always been a big proponent of persistence; some would instead prefer to describe what I do as borderline annoying. But a week went by, then two of paying for my spot in the dorm room, and the $1,000 did not seem like so much after all. The third week Alfrede had the most fantastic news I could have heard. I would become her dishwasher. I could run the pots and pans machine. It was a great job because I worked 6:30 to 9:30 p.m. only. That meant I never had to work during ski hours, which was not true of any other ski bum jobs.

The deal included room and board, a season pass, and $100 per month spending money. Plus, I would get one day off every week. I was sure I didn't need a day off, but that was Alfrede's standard deal. She pointed out that I might want to get out of the canyon occasionally, as "canyon phobia" became a syndrome for many of her workers over a long season. I felt like I had died and gone to heaven.

My new (free) room was in the original old wooden lodge built in the 1930s, now converted into employee housing. A room that held three people was the size of a large closet. The beds were built into one wall like bunk beds with drawers under them. The other long wall had a sink, a mirror, and a few more built-in drawers. The short wall across from the door had one large picture window looking out at the slopes. A shared boy's bathroom was just down the hall, like in a dormitory. It was about as clean as a dorm bathroom, too.

I skied one hundred days straight that season. That's right, one hundred days of Utah powder. I was focused. I had to figure out how to get the turn on my outside edge (the left edge of my single left ski) to be symmetrical to the turn on my inside edge. That was the big nut to crack; that and pure strength and endurance. The other ski bums couldn't understand why I went out even on bad days. They went out only on powder days or on those beautiful few days right after a big storm, of which there weren't many that year. The 1976-77 winter still ranks as one of the worst snow droughts in Alta history.

I didn't care. I just needed enough snow to keep working on that outside edge turn. Skiing every single day improved my skills quickly. That's what motivated me. That's why I went out every day—even poor ski days—when saner ski bums stayed back in the lodge. I drew attention. I got to know everyone who worked on the mountain. One person who sought me out and took a real interest in me was Paul Norm, the assistant director of the ski school. Paul had had seven concussions growing up as a ski racer, and his head, neck, and spine hurt whenever they were jarred. So he had to ski very smoothly out of self-defense. He had perfected a beautiful, smooth style, where his head and shoulders didn't move at all, even when he skied the bumps. He went down the bumps very fast with his feet and knees pumping and steering hard, but his upper body was smooth and quiet. I was fooled into thinking he was not going that fast, but he was. He was exactly the model of skier I wanted to become.

Paul liked the idea of teaching amputee skiing, and had tried one-legged skiing as a challenge a few times. He decided to make me his pet project. He configured a contraption for the back of his left binding to hold his unused right foot behind his skiing leg. It was like a little basket sticking off the back of his mounted binding where he could put the toe of his free foot. It looked like he was water skiing with that foot back there. This put him in the position of an amputee skier as accurately as a two-legger could be. He even found a pair of outriggers.

None of the ski instructors were very busy that season due to the poor conditions. Paul and I skied a lot together, and for free he gave me a private lesson two or three times a week. We'd work on staying still and smooth through the bumps, skiing powder when we could find it, and, most of all, performing completely symmetrical left- and right-carved turns.

After many weeks of this, Paul paid me the ultimate compliment, indicating I had in fact already achieved my goal. He asked me to team-teach carved turning classes with him. I couldn't believe it. He was asking me, an amputee, to teach skiing to two-legged students. And it was not for beginners' classes. It was for his advanced carved turning classes. His reasoning was that he was tired of two-legged skiers learning to carve their turns continually asking him on which ski their weight should be. That is the wrong question in carving. It's all about edges and knees, not the weighting. With me teaching and demonstrating, he knew none of the students could possibly ask which ski to weight; instead, they would have to focus on watching the edges like he wanted them to. It was an honor and it was fun. Suddenly I was in the spotlight *for my skiing*. For someone worried if I'd ever even ski just three short years ago, this was a hugely satisfying and dramatic moment.

The other person in the ski school with whom I spent a lot of time was its founder and director, Alf Engen. Alf was in his late 70s and still skied beautifully. He had been a Norwegian champion in the 1932 Olympics. He said he loved skiing with me because I was a smooth, fast skier and because I was fearless. With Paul and Alf as skiing friends, with getting to teach and having ski patrol know me by name and offer me free skis when they broke half of a pair, with getting darkly tanned, and with making great friends with all the other ski bums, Alta was heaven for me. I never thought about my future or if I even had a future. I was living—really living—day-to-day. And that was enough for me.

By all rights, my brain should have rotted during that winter. I never read anything more than trail signs that entire season. When not skiing, washing pots, or sleeping, I was playing foosball in the bar, drinking beer, or just hanging out with other employees. There was a lot of pot, a lot of cocaine, a lot of hookups, and all Jimmy Buffet all the time. I was one of the few not partaking of the pot and coke (or hookups), but the beer I was happy to imbibe. I still did not like pot because I hated to put smoke into my lungs. Besides, I told myself, "It's just medicine to stop nausea, right?" Cocaine scared me, and I refused to put it up my nose, period.

I stuck with beer and wine. A couple of times, I had too much beer and wine. I learned the misery of a force five hangover. A particularly nasty one was so bad that it took thirty minutes to sit up, another thirty minutes to put on my sock (luckily I didn't need to put on a second one), and hours before I could get showered and dressed. The experience reminded me how distressingly similar the effect of chemotherapy was to a bad hangover, and I vowed to avoid them in the future.

Many sunny afternoons after skiing, we all climbed out of the dormitory with wine and cheese, and of course Jimmy Buffet, onto the angled roof where no one on the mountain could see us, and we stripped down to sunbathe nude. It was a gigantic step for me to get naked in front of other people, but they were all completely used to seeing me one-legged. I hoped they would not mind seeing my stump, which is not very attractive. I still felt behind my age group when it came to girls, so I appreciated seeing those very beautiful girls without clothes on. They were all quite attached, however, so looking was all I got to do.

I learned the mountain like the back of my hand. Alta didn't have trail signs on all the slopes, and few slopes were cut through trees and easily visible. Their slogan was, "Alta is for skiers" but perhaps it should have been "Alta is for locals." A certain face of a large buttress would have a name that was not listed anywhere, yet was a well-known trail to locals. "Yellow Trail," "Gunsight," "West Rustler," "Stonecrusher," and "Eagle's Nest" were like that, with nary a sign anywhere on the mountain. It was not easy to get to any of the best runs at Alta. High-speed, long, bone-rattling bumpy traverses, climbing—sometimes with, sometimes without skis—picking through rocks at trail entrances, or a combination of all three were typical of skiing at Alta.

I had to learn how to slow down on a narrow traverse using a substitute for the two-legger snowplow. It was important that I build up strength to last on the high-speed, very bumpy and rutted, mile-long high traverses. These traverses went out along major buttress formations that were characteristic of Alta. One formed the Rustler set of runs. Alf's High Rustler, the furthest one out, was consistently listed as one of North America's top ten most difficult runs. I tried to do it once a day if it was open. I only did significant climbs with skis off if I was with someone who would carry my ski while I used the outriggers as crutches. Since the outriggers were made of crutches attached to little skis, and since skis are meant to slide across snow, this was always a hair-raising experience. Getting the little ski tips to act like climbing crutches required a huge effort, and these climbs were much more exhausting for me than for two-leggers hiking by foot. On even a modest climb, I would get tired, sweaty, and out of breath. Not all climbs required skis to come off, and many I would do the same way I skied most of the time: alone. Climbing is how to get to late powder, and it's how to get to where there are no people; it's where Alta hides its best skiing. So, since it was hard even for two-leggers, I was on it.

This was a low snow year the entire season, not just at its late start. The snow was so thin that there were a lot of rocks, and I badly damaged several skis. Luckily, the ski patrol did, too, and they kept giving me the other half of a pair whenever they destroyed one. I think they enjoyed my attitude, and it was no skin off their backs to give me a single ski when they broke one of their own. It was just going into the trash otherwise. It never occurred to me that during the course of a one-hundred-day season I might burn my ski out even if I didn't bang it up mercilessly on rocks. Thankfully, the ski patrol provided me with an endless supply.

The most dramatic destruction of one of my skis was when I sped over a rise and found myself heading straight into a field of jagged rocks. There was no way to go around them. I was committed, and there was no room or time for me to stop. All I could do was brace myself, sit back, hit the field of jagged rocks, and try not to get too banged up. When it was over and I got up, I was surprisingly undamaged. But my edges were completely sprung out to the sides, extending one foot from each side of the ski. I was not going anywhere with a ski looking like that; I had no choice but to wait for the ski patrol. When one showed up, I asked if I could borrow one of his skis and we would each ski down on one, but he wouldn't go for that plan. Plan B put me into his toboggan. The patrolman was psyched because he could go fast and not worry about jostling a passenger who was in no way injured. He never got to do that except with an empty toboggan. For me it was quite a ride at amazing speed. The toboggan and I were two feet off the snow at many points on the way down. Once down the mountain, and with my ruined ski safely in the trash, I had a whole building full of ski patrollers thrusting skis on me. I lost almost no time getting back up on the mountain.

I was still frustrated at how much strength and endurance I required from my one leg to ski well and for long periods, especially since I was always drawn to steep mogul runs. Early on, I pushed myself past the burning leg sensation to the next level of fatigue, when my leg began to shake just before it reached total collapse. Then I found myself in a heap in the snow with my leg cramping. The cure for this was skiing every day for weeks and weeks. Eventually, I was strong enough that I could ski all day on one leg and not be exhausted. Fatigue when skiing has remained a lifelong challenge. I have tried stair-hopping, rope-jumping, biking, special ski and weight machines, but no simulated exercise exactly matches skiing. Unless and until I can make time to ski more like forty to fifty days per year, I will have a challenge to ski past the point in the day when all my two-legged ski companions give up.

When you have only one leg, it gets no rest. Even when stopped on the trail or in the lift line, the normal side-to-side shifting two-leggers do is not possible for me. The only relief I get is from using the outriggers like crutches to take some weight off my leg. Alta lift operators decided that amputee skiers should not wait in lift lines and should enter through the ski school line. That proved to be a godsend for me, allowing a modicum of extra rest by getting me on the chair lifts a little sooner. I watched all the two-leggers wait thirty or forty minutes, while I skipped the lift line and rode up so I could rest and get back on the slope sooner. On a busy weekend day, I undoubtedly skied a good thirty percent more than the two-leggers I bypassed in lift lines.

April came, the snow melted, and I had to come out of my state of ski bum bliss and think about what came next. I hadn't thought this far ahead. I didn't think I needed to. My first simple observations were that the snow was gone and I was not dead. *Now what?*

The obvious thing to me was to try to follow in Paul Norm's boot steps and see if it was possible to become a ski instructor. Why not? He'd shown me that it was possible—he and those students in his carved turn class. When I suggested this to him, he didn't laugh at me. He said he would write a letter of reference and make some introductions. Alf also wrote a strong letter I could use to get past people's initial skepticism. I wanted to head back home first but keep the option open of pursuing the challenge of becoming the first-ever professional amputee ski instructor.

I checked in with my parents, with whom I had not communicated much, and it just so happened they were about to head off for a late-season ski week in Quebec. They told me if I wanted to race home, I could join them. Well, I wanted. In no way was I sick of skiing. I just needed somewhere that had snow.

To make it in time required driving thirty-two hours straight, all the way to Detroit. Then, if I made it, I would climb in their car for a twenty-two-hour drive to Mt. Tremblant. I made it by using No-Doz, coffee, cold air, and many self-inflicted face slaps. I drove all through the night and arrived home just two hours before they were to depart. That is one ski-trip drive with my family that I do not remember; I slept soundly the entire way. I got in that one last ski trip to end the season at the place where I first tried to ski on one leg just four seasons before. I had made a lot of progress since then.

I was still alive, so I could think of nothing better to do than to finish college. Not the most auspicious rationale for a college education. All I had left was two quarters on campus and I would be off to junior year abroad as a senior, as promised to me. So I went back for spring and summer quarters, picking up where I had left off. Because I had gone eight quarters straight my freshman and sophomore years, when I went off to Alta, I had been a full two quarters ahead of my peer group of other juniors. So even after spending two quarters ski bumming, I was not behind. It seemed too good to be true to go from skiing for six months at Alta to six months in France with full college credits. I might have thought I had died and gone to heaven . . . if I wasn't so happy not to have died.

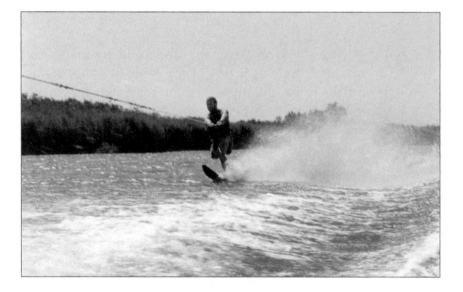

FIVE

NORMAL SCHNORMAL

To be normal is the aim of the unsuccessful.

— Carl Gustav Jung, psychiatrist

Normal is not something to aspire to; it's something to get away from.

— Jodie Foster, movie actress

The only normal people are the one's you don't know very well.

— Alfred Adler, psychologist

Certainly losing a leg was traumatic, and knowing that cancer had been—and might still be—in my body was horrifying. But what hurt the most initially was the feeling that I suddenly had no friends because I wasn't a "normal" teenager anymore. In my case, normal was violently ripped away from me. With some people, normal is something they are born "outside of." That is an important distinction because when the change happens later in life, it can make the adjustment harder; it seems like you lost something you had before. But in the end, in terms of how society treats you and makes you feel, it's the same. You are simply not normal. Back then, I didn't want to be different, and I didn't want to be placed in a group that was separate from everyone else. Yet, the last thing I wanted to do was join a support group of other amputees. I rebelled against the words disabled and handicapped. I didn't even consider getting a handicapped-parking placard for the first five years. I rejected having those labels placed on me then, and still don't think of myself in those terms today—nor do people who know me. When someone becomes disabled, all he initially wants to be is normal again. The changes in his life make him feel inadequate because it *seems* he can no longer do things that he did before. *Seems* is a key word here. As I discovered over time, I could find a way to do most of the things I thought I could not do. With some, like skiing, I would eventually do much better than I had ever done back when I was "normal." Dependency is another reason you strive to get back to normal. It doesn't feel good to be dependent on others for things you used to do for yourself. Independence and self-reliance are the first steps toward removing the overpowering obsession with getting back to normal.

But what is normal? When we say someone is normal, we are

saying that person does not stand out; that person is not deviant. If you are normal, you don't draw attention, unless or until you want to. If you are normal, you are able to participate; you are able to be competitive. But normal is not always a positive thing. Celebrities and other highly public figures bemoan the difficulty they have in leading a *normal* life or providing a *normal* childhood to their kids. Society uses normal as a weapon against individuals who are outside some physical and/or behavioral limits of acceptability. This is especially difficult for teenagers. They are already highly susceptible to a strong need to fit in. Acceptance, friends, and being part of the group are powerful forces for teenagers as part of their normal development and socialization.

Disability has many negatives in society. For people disabled due to a missing body part, a prosthesis removes the obvious physical differences on which people focus. People cannot see that you are physically different, so you can interact with them more normally. It's as if the elephant has left the room. Getting stared at is never comfortable; it is a constant reminder you are different and don't fit in. For those who have a deformity, who are in a wheelchair, or who have some undisguisable condition, there is no relief from the staring. Children can be pretty harsh and cruel to anyone who looks different. When I was sixteen and had just had an amputation, because they found out it was from cancer, my friends headed for the hills. I was completely shunned. In 1973, some people even thought you could catch cancer. But today many kids still shun peers with almost any disease because it makes that person different and because anything hinting at death is too scary to face. Today, little kids seem to think if you are missing a leg or have some other physically striking difference, the disability must affect your hearing. Walking on the pool deck, I constantly hear little kids yelling to their friends or their parents, "What happened to that man's leg?" They think I am deaf, as well as walking on crutches. Individuals turn that on themselves when they feel inadequate. Jane Smith writes in *Trying to be Normal,* "The most difficult part of being disabled is coming to terms with the negative values I have internalized. I am disabled and I am trying to work through my prejudices about my own disability and others. My gut reaction was to deny that I had these feelings, but denial does not allow me to come to terms with my devaluing prejudices."

Once you feel like you have "come back," for many if not most, there is suddenly this transformation into striving for supernormal. In my case, once I felt like I had more or less achieved my goal of "normal," I began to strive for what you might call "overachiev-ing" and exceeding what people thought was possible for me. This behavior was actually—well—normal. When knocked down hard, we will try to come back and exceed normal. Lance Armstrong, Michael J. Fox, and Stephen Hawking are well-known examples of this, but hundreds of thousands of people whose names you don't know are equally obsessed with doing the impossible.

For the disabled person who comes back, the goal changes from striving to be normal to striving to be better, at least in one small slice of life. This starts by finding something you can do. It doesn't matter what it is. It could be cards; it could be a sport; it could be an intellectual pursuit. Disabled people are highly motivated and will pour everything they have into that "something" they find. They focus; they work hard; they put everything into excelling, and suddenly they find they are going beyond their able-bodied counterparts. For me, this sent me into risk-taking territory. Once I excelled beyond what two-leggers could do in one area, I wanted to push the limits in other areas. Why? Mostly because someone said, "I bet you can't do that." Whenever I heard that, I responded big time.

Where does this fight come from? People often ask me if the personality trait to be a fighter was there before I lost my leg. I can't be sure, but I don't think it was because I never really stood out before. I was born during a major flood in California's central valley in the summer of 1956 while my dad was working as a surgeon on an Air Force base. When I was just two weeks old, we moved to St. Louis for Dad's surgery residency (which he had put on hold for the war). We lived there for four years. After Dad finished his residency, when I was four, we moved to Syracuse, New York, so that he could start a private practice. We lived on a very long steep hill behind the university. The top of the hill was a huge circular roadway that was part of a park, with trees and long grass all around it. We lived in a large, grey wooden house a little ways down the hill, with a huge terraced backyard adjacent to thick woods traversed by an intricate network of well-worn paths.

My brother, Michael, was three and a half years older than me. Sometimes we played together, but most of the time he and his buddies ditched me as the annoying, bratty, younger brother. I remember chasing them around a lot in an effort to be part of their group. Many of those chases ended with me getting hurt. I frequently crashed into the corner of the house where a wooden molding stuck out especially far, right at the level of my head. I busted my head open so often on that wooden molding that Dad stopped stitching me up and just used butterfly Band-Aids to stop the bleeding.

My first resilience test occurred when I broke my leg at the age of six. We were skiing at a local mountain near Syracuse. It was my second year skiing, and I broke my right leg because I was snow plowing, got stuck in wet, deep snow, and did a slow twisting fall. I remember the fall vividly. It all happened in slow motion. I was near the lift on nearly flat ground. My skis were buried in the heavy snow. I lost my balance, but as I was in a snowplow position (ski tips tightly together, ski heels spread widely apart forming a wedge), I didn't just fall to the side. I fell toward the ski tips, twisting my lower right leg as I went down. As I was going down, I felt a twinge of pain and then I heard a crack. That's when the pain got very intense. I started crying and screaming. I couldn't move. I was all twisted up. Ski patrol came quickly, freed my feet, fixed me up with a splint, and put me into a toboggan for a ride to the infirmary. They called my parents over the resort-wide PA system. Dad says he never skied so fast in his life and probably didn't make a single turn all the way down from the top of the hill. It was the same leg that would cause much bigger problems for me many years later.

I was in a full leg cast for a broken tibia. We decorated the cast with lots of cool drawings. As a six-year-old, I found getting around on crutches to be very tricky. I had this huge dead weight to swing around. Stairs were especially scary. It felt like I was close to tumbling face first every time I had to go down them. When I got back to my first grade class on crutches, one of my fun-loving classmates decided to try the old pull-the-chair-out trick right as I sat down. I earned a bruised tailbone and he earned a day home from school.

I wasn't very willing to be sedentary with my cast on once the pain subsided. I managed to get up to the top of our long, steep hill with my red Radio Flyer wagon. It just seemed like the thing to do to ride down that hill on the wagon, cast be damned. I shot down at breakneck speed, or should I say "break-cast" speed. I started to have trouble keeping the wagon stable, and it kept going faster and faster until I hit a tree and the wagon rolled over. I wasn't hurt badly, but when I looked down, I saw that the cast had completely unwound from my leg and was in pieces all around me. The babysitter called Dad home from his surgery office. He wasn't very happy with me, but he took me to the orthopedist to get a new cast put on.

A few weeks later, now in cast number two, I jumped into a full bathtub to discover that plaster melts in water. Another trip to the doctor. Dad was pretty pissed off at me by this point. Now in cast number three, I fell down the stairs and it shattered again. I didn't do it on purpose, but I still thought it was funny. Little kids practically have plastic bones, and luckily I healed completely in six weeks. Who knows what else I might have tried if it had taken longer. Many years later, my dad broke the same bone, and it took more than six months in a cast for his forty-something-year-old leg to heal. But then, he never rode down the hill in his wagon or jumped in a bathtub with his cast.

I had a temper and wouldn't allow myself to be pushed beyond a certain point. Like any kid, I had limited ways to deal with this. So once, when I really snapped, I ended up breaking every window in my room. My room was an old screened-in porch where all the screens had been converted into windows. This room had probably eight or ten windows, each with top and bottom panes. For reasons long since forgotten, I got really upset at my dad. Once alone in my room, I took off my belt and started swinging it, buckle end out, over my head like a cowboy with a lasso. Then I started walking around the room hitting every pane of glass with the buckle. I loved the sound of the breaking glass, and soon I totally lost any sense of what I was doing. As I shattered each window, I released a little more of my anger until finally it was spent. Or at least there were no more windows to shatter. I looked around in shock at what I had done. Glass was everywhere. The concept of consequences started to seep into my consciousness, and I was fearful about what would happen to me next.

Dad came running up the stairs with fire in his eyes. His look scared me. He grabbed me by the arm, sat on the stairs, threw me face down on his knee, and just started swatting my behind as hard as he could. It hurt a lot. I screamed and struggled to get away, but he was too strong. Now I was even madder at him. Confined to my room, my anger again grew, but I no longer had any windows on which to expend it.

Like all kids in second grade, I loved to climb trees. We had elaborate hide-and-seek games. Tree climbing was an effective strategy, especially up in the more densely foliated trees. One tree I loved was the Hoke's apple tree next door, out of which I managed to fall. I lost my grip up near the top of that tree and fell straight down fifteen feet, managing to land flat on my back, probably saving me from a broken back or worse.

When I was entering the third grade, we moved to Birmingham, a northwest suburb of Detroit. Detroit sits on a river, actually a strait, which connects Lake St. Claire to Lake Erie and separates the United States from Canada. Detroit names many of the main roads sequentially as mile roads. Detroit's northern city limit is 8 Mile Road. Birmingham is between 14 and 17 Mile Roads. We lived near 15 Mile Road.

Our neighborhood was right next to the huge Seaholm High School campus, which included my school, Midvale Elementary. Neighboring a school meant easy access to baseball diamonds, a full track, a football field, and the usual playgrounds associated with an elementary school. We used all those fields a lot for playing pickup games of baseball, touch football, dog ball throwing, Frisbee tossing, kite flying, and more.

After third grade at Midvale, I switched to the Brookside private school, which is part of the Cranbrook complex in Bloomfield Hills. Brookside is the elementary school, after which the girls go to Kingswood and the boys go to Cranbrook for junior high and high school. There is also an art school, an art museum, a science museum, and many gardens on the palatial campus of Cranbrook. As in many schools, the kids at Brookside had to recite the Pledge of Allegiance at the start of each day and before assemblies. I didn't believe in God and wasn't willing to be told I should by anybody, including adults. My obstinacy led to an early lesson about determination, about being willing to be different, and about sticking to my guns.

I refused to say the Pledge because it required me to say "under God." Since I didn't believe in those words, I was unwilling to say them. I was so hardcore about this that I wouldn't even stand up when others were reciting it. No one told me to do this. My parents had no knowledge I was so steadfast in my refusal. That refusal got me sent to the office. Mind you, I was a good student and I never got into trouble, so I rarely frequented the office. But rules were rules, so off I went. Much to the school's surprise—and to mine—my parents backed me up. I think they were impressed that their ten-year-old kid had conviction about some issue. That turned into an officially school-sanctioned exemption from having to participate in the Pledge of Allegiance. For the first time in my young life, I felt completely vindicated. I liked the feeling of being different, of being singled out. I especially liked the fact that I had just proven that if I felt really strongly about something, and was willing to stand my ground, I could prevail.

Ice skating is the winter thing to do when you live in Michigan. There were lots of local rinks and backyard rinks during the winter season. We played backyard hockey. I never took to it seriously, but I loved the speed I could achieve on the ice, and I loved being good at something physical and difficult. As members of the Cranbook community, we could use the Cranbook ice skating rink.

As I became interested in girls, I discovered this was a good way to spend time with them. Well, in a weird, twelve-year-old sort of way it was. We boys would skate around the rink fast and accidentally/on purpose bump the girls as we went by. Bumping into them, or spraying them with ice while showing our prowess at high-speed hockey stops, was our early adolescent way of showing our interest. It was also great to interact with them in the warming hut and have hot chocolate during breaks from high-speed girl bumping.

Sailing became a summer family passion. We had a Sunfish:

a wonderful, fun little boat that we could carry on top of the car. It was perfect on small Michigan lakes, but over time we pushed the boundaries of where we would take it. My dad was a fearless sailor, and he made sure to instill that in me. He had little access to outdoor activities as a kid, growing up as a city-dweller with childhood asthma in the Bronx. He learned to ski and sail as an adult and became passionate about those activities. Dad passed on to me his drive and fearlessness, attributes that became critical in my life as events unfolded.

As kids, we had to prove we could solo sail in our local little Orchard Lake by taking our Sunfish out, tipping it over, and single-handedly righting it. That took a certain amount of raw weight combined with some finesse. I was twelve before I could finally do it. I worked and worked at it. But for a long time I was just not heavy enough. When I finally succeeded, I was so proud that I wanted to do it all the time, not only to prove myself to my dad and the others, but also to prove myself to me. Now I had a very precious privilege: I was trusted to sail the boat completely alone. It was the first "alone" thing I really wanted to do and had sought with focus and determination.

Like lots of families, we went to different places for a vacation week every summer. Our favorite place of all was way up in Ontario on Lake Temagami. *Temagami* is a Native American word that means "deep water by the shore." Many areas reach more than fifty feet deep within twenty feet of shore. At its deepest, it is 750 feet, and it is huge. Formed by a glacier, it has many north/south oriented, glacier-scoured fingers that create more than three thousand miles of shoreline. That includes the shoreline of its 1,250 islands. From space it looks like the body of a giant spider with outstretched legs.

We stayed several summers in a little cabin on Rabbit Nose Island in the middle of the lake. Rabbit Nose is accessible only by boat. The taxi boat came and got us at the beginning of the week, towing our Sunfish along behind it.

There were many activities on Rabbit Nose Island and they had many different kinds of boats there, including canoes. I was not terribly interested in the canoe until Dad told me about gunneling, something he learned not while growing up in the Bronx, but at summer camp, where he worked as a counselor. To gunnel a canoe, you stand on the gunnels (the top edge of the canoe's sides) near the back end of the canoe. After you get balanced on the gunnels, you start pumping your legs up and down, which makes the canoe start to spurt ahead on the waves you create, like squeezing a watermelon seed between your fingers. As you get the rhythm going, you can pump harder and harder to go fast and far. Native Americans actually used this technique to quietly cross a body of water with a bow and arrow in their hands, sneaking up on their target along the shore—something not possible if their hands were busy paddling. First, I spent hours just getting enough balance to gunnel at all—with lots of dramatic falls into the very cold lake. Then I aimed to perfect my technique, with a goal of gunnelling long distances. I had to get really good at it because Dad said it was hard and that few could get it right. I decided that I had to be the best at it. Even back then, Dad had a way of challenging me that made me strive to be the best. It took focus and a willingness to forgo lots of other activities in lieu of learning this hard task. Eventually I was the best of anyone on the island because my obsession drove me to spend the necessary hours perfecting it. Once I was good at something difficult, I loved to show off doing it. Especially if it was something that my brother, Michael, couldn't do. I would gunnel for miles if I was allowed to.

Early on, another important part of summer for me was staying at my grandmother's. I was her favorite. All my cousins thought I was nuts to want to be with her at all. They considered a two-week stay with Grandmother the second worst punishment in the world. Second only to a stay in a Soviet Gulag. She had quite an estate in Sudbury, Massachusetts, which my mother had never been able to enjoy, as they had moved there just as she went off to Wellesley College. It has since been donated to the Audubon Society. She had a pond, a tennis court, a barn, and fields of sheep and ducks. I could spend hours exploring behind the pond, in the backfields, or across the road in the barn where the farm animals lived. I claimed the one ram they kept in a separate field as my own pet. I creatively named him "Rammy." While I considered Rammy to be my pet, he did not have reciprocal warm feelings toward me and would chase and butt me if I tried to set foot on his field.

The other vicious little creatures that chased me were the geese.

Farmyard geese are not the docile creatures you might expect, and I had many pecking injuries from my interactions just trying to feed them.

I helped to install a space trolley between two huge oak trees next to the tennis court. I often raced back and forth, hanging from a short rope ladder that was attached to a pulley that rolled across two taut wires suspended between the trees. I spent hours by myself on that space trolley, imagining space adventures, seeing how fast and how long I could push myself back and forth. Mostly my goal for the week with Granny was making money. She was tough, but she paid well. I would weed the garden, do small repairs, walk the dogs, feed Rammy and his harem, as well as the scary geese. From the financial perspective of a preteen, I could make a fortune.

Summer life with Granny was extremely regimented. Afternoon ginger ale and ginger snap cookies were served at four o'clock on the back patio. No other drinks. No other cookies. No other time. No other place. She kept three full-sized poodles and a very rare and very expensive type of Siamese cat, which she had declawed and neutered. The dogs hated the cat, so we had to keep the two species completely separate at all costs. Many years and several generations of Siamese cats later, Granny became forgetful and sometimes left the cat locked in the basement, where it had to fend for itself for three or more days. Eventually the cat became too much for her and she was about to have it put down. I was married with kids by then, and we took the cat off her hands, even though we did not much favor cats. That cat was psychotic. But after an intense year of kindness and patience, he regained his sanity and became the most affectionate and loving cat to us and to our dogs.

Either it was innate in my personality or I learned very early to be adaptable even with difficult situations and difficult people like Granny. I learned that by adapting, I actually got more of what I wanted. Most others, including all my siblings and cousins who refused to adapt to Granny's unreasonable ways, were left behind and were poorer for it. Another early lesson that I have never forgotten is that if a goal is important, do whatever it takes to achieve it.

Summers were not just family trips, lawn jobs, and visiting Grandmother. I developed an infatuation with summer camp early on and became the one in the family addicted to spending more and more time there. I went mostly to YMCA camps that offered canoeing throughout Michigan. Another summer I went to a sailing camp on Lake Huron, where I took my sailing skills to the next level. One camp was a truck travel camp. All we did was ride over Michigan's two peninsulas in the back of a truck—seeing all kinds of cool and not-so-cool things—sleeping out under the stars every night.

My summer camp career peaked and ended at Camp Mongotassee. It was here that I was given a challenge, focused on it, achieved it, and did so beyond what anyone else ever had. Mongotassee was the gold standard in summer YMCA camps. They had an elite leadership program with three levels: Hunter, Warrior, and Medicine Lodge. You had to try out for each level and could make it to a new level only once per year. So at minimum, it took three years to make it all the way to the top. Very few ever made it to Medicine Lodge, and no one had ever gotten there in only three years. It was a challenge, and it was a good way to be accepted and even admired, so I went for it with a vengeance. It was hard work, and they put me through a lot to get to the next level. But I made it all the way to Medicine Lodge in a record three years. It gave me many privileges, like a special table at dinner, fewer tent inspections, less supervision as we walked around camp, and free access to the lake and the boats. The other campers respected my achievement and looked up to me. It was the biggest achievement of my life to that point.

Back in Birmingham, we rode our bikes everywhere, including to the schoolyard to play touch football. We also rode to the local quickie mart to get the latest comic books and candy bars. When I was about fourteen, I fell off my bike while chasing my older brother across the front yard. That resulted in a broken thumb and having my right arm put in a cast. I had to learn how to write with my left hand, a skill I was able to maintain for the rest of my life and which was of great convenience when I became a professor. (Writing on a chalkboard left to right, as we do in English, works much better with the left hand because one's body stays out of the way of the students behind you trying to read the board.) The broken thumb didn't hurt much, and I could use the casted arm as a club, which was a lot of fun when dealing with my troublesome brother who caused the accident in the first place.

When I was in sixth grade and close to graduating from Brook-side, my parents took just me out to dinner. Something big was up. This had never happened before, so I knew it couldn't be good news. I was right: they announced that I wouldn't be attending junior and high school at Cranbrook with all my friends. The problem was money. They explained to me that they believed the younger kids needed the good start provided by a private elementary school—just like I had had—but that once a solid base was established, we would all do fine in public school. Rationalization perhaps, but I understood the limited financial resources available. I also understood fairness when it came to my younger siblings.

I was apprehensive of the new school. Covington Junior High was a sprawling, one-story, cream-colored modern school about a mile and a half from our house. The main hallways had little alcoves that housed our tall lockers. The contrast to the old brick and wood, warm and welcoming Brookside could not have been greater. I carried around my chosen musical instrument, a viola. Knowing no one and carrying around an instrument set me apart from the kids with ready-made cliques brought with them from their respective elementary schools. This forced me to rely on myself—a skill that would prove invaluable.

At Covington, shop class started out as a drafting class, which I really enjoyed. I designed, drew, and then finally learned how to build speaker cabinets that were part of my master plan for a top-notch stereo. The machines in shop class were very scary to me. I was petrified of losing a body part. I finished the speaker cabinets, and they were strong but not pretty. Then, from my little catalog, I bought the speaker components after which I had been lusting for so long that the catalog was crumpled, faded, and soggy from pocket sweat. It looked like a message that arrived in a bottle. Now I had speakers, but nothing to put sound in them for a year. They just sat there as I stared at them longingly.

Two summers of lawn jobs allowed me to order the Heathkit stereo components. I sat down and learned how to solder so I could build them from a kit. My prior experience at close kit-like work had just been puzzles, plastic model cars and spaceships, and model sailing ships. I didn't know a resistor or transistor from a model car fender, but I followed directions religiously. When completed, I had by far the best stereo of anyone my age.

Playing the viola had a dark side that I could not have anticipated. As I started junior high, I was short for my age, plus I still had a little lingering baby fat and a few effeminate traits that were highlighted by carrying around the viola. All of this, on top of being the new kid and knowing no one, led to major harassment. The first year was miserable. The most common epithet thrown at me was "fag." The boys formed two major groups of greasers and jocks, and both harassed me. Of course, there were boys that were in neither group, but I guess they didn't care much what I did. I cared and the harassment bothered me. I wanted to be accepted; I wanted to be in a group. During the summer between seventh and eighth grade, I was determined to do something about it, but it was actually nature that did the most. I grew a full six inches that summer. I also bought some weights and used them extensively. The baby fat had disappeared. I gained a lot of weight, most of it muscle, and I dropped the viola like a hot potato.

Back at school, the first kid that dared to call me a "fag" was not too smart and certainly lacked a keen sense of the obvious. I was ready for this. I had changed in more than just physical ways. I popped him hard and fast with one quick right jab and broke his nose. Amazingly, I didn't even get in trouble because it happened nowhere near school grounds. It stopped the teasing in its tracks, never to occur again. I never again hit someone with my fist. One more lesson learned. I could change if I wanted and needed to. I could fight back and win when directly challenged. I was becoming stronger, and I was gaining self-confidence. Good, because, boy was I about to need it.

The swim team became the replacement for the viola. It became my key to being fully accepted, becoming part of a group, and gaining people's respect. It was also something that got the attention of girls, and that was getting increasingly important to me.

Coach Denny was the gym teacher as well as the swim coach. He was a very gruff guy. Even though his day job was teaching, his heart was clearly with coaching. He created a swim section of gym class partly so he could scout for swimmers to join his team. During that swim section, he was actually holding swim team tryouts. He picked me as someone with potential. I guess all those weekends of

YMCA swim classes that my parents signed me up for had paid off. I had enjoyed swimming at the Y and, like all things I got involved with, worked hard to try to be the best at it. When Coach Denny told me I was good enough to join the swim team, I was beside myself. Of course I would join, I told him. And I would work hard.

Coach Denny coached my junior high team as if we were already in high school. We had four thousand-yard workouts every day after school. That's 160 lengths of the pool, which took a solid two hours to swim. This was before goggles were invented. No one wore eye protection in those days, and being a school pool with lots of bodies in it, they used a hefty dose of chlorine. After four thousand yards in chlorine, none of us could see at all. It was impossible to read, and I couldn't even watch TV. My eyes stung badly every night, but by morning they were ready to be traumatized again after school.

After swim practice each evening, it was so late that there were no buses running. I had to walk the mile and a half home every night. Swim team is a winter sport, so it was dark and cold. Many nights my hair froze solid by the time I got home. All the way home, lights looked like diffused, glowing blobs, but my eyes were mostly closed anyway because they stung too much to keep them open.

I became one of the fastest swimmers on the team. I was a sprinter specializing in the fifty-yard free as well as the free and medley relays. Ultimately, along with my teammates, I held the state record in both relays for a number of years. I was a very nervous competitor, perhaps because I required myself to be the best and to win. I put most of the pressure on myself, but Coach Denny added plenty himself. I couldn't sleep before a meet. When it was time to race, I started shaking up on the starting blocks. In crucial meets, after Coach would say something wondrously helpful like, "The team can win but only if you win your event; it's all up to you now," I would totally miss the wall on a flip turn and blow the event and the entire meet. Something had to give, and in my case it was my gastrointestinal tract. As an eighth grader, I actually got an ulcer. That meant I had to eat Maalox tablets, drink gallons of milk, and eat lots of peanut butter sandwiches. I loved swim practice. I loved the camaraderie. I loved the attention I was getting. I just couldn't handle the swim meets. In ninth grade I had to back out of a couple of meets because of the ulcer.

Math teachers have a stereotype of being somewhat eccentric. In Covington, the geometry teacher may even have helped establish that stereotype. When class started in the fall, he never even cared to learn our names. Instead, he just gave us number assignments for the row and column of our assigned seat in the class in a math formulation, called a tuple, written (x,y). I was $(4,5)$ which, strangely enough, I have never forgotten. At the beginning of each class, he called out the tuple for people to go to the board and do the homework assignment in front of the whole class. While you were working on problems on the chalkboard, he would walk back and forth right behind you, ominously carrying the textbook. If you got the problem wrong, he whacked you on the back of the head with his book. He hit the boys he didn't like pretty hard. But he never actually hit me. Luckily, whenever he called out for Mr. $(4,5)$ to go to the board, I was fortunate—or maybe he was—that I always got the problems right.

Skiing was a major part of our family life during the winter. Besides our little local club with just a rope tow and ninety-second-long runs, every year we took a weeklong Christmas trip way up into Canada, north of Montreal, to Mt. Tremblant. We stayed in a family cabin at the bottom of the mountain. These were cozy cabins with separate bedrooms for older boys, the little kids, and parents, as well as a great room with a fireplace. We had to walk a few hundred yards to the big lodge for breakfast and dinner each day. No big deal, unless it was twenty below zero, which it often was. At that temperature, it was so cold the moisture in your nose would freeze and you could feel your nose crackle. Some days it remained that cold all day. Twenty below, not counting wind chill at the bottom, meant thirty or even forty below up on the mountain, and especially on the lifts. They had a serious safety concern on days this cold and issued big "lift coats" to put over our ski clothing to protect us when riding up the mountain. At the top, they required everyone to go right into the warming hut to avoid frostbite. Once warmed up, we skied down, stopping to look at each other's faces for white patches. If one of us had a patch, another took a hand out of its glove and warmed that person's face with it. Now the hand was at risk, so it went inside a jacket under an armpit to warm up before being put back into the glove. At the bottom, everyone was so cold we went into the warming hut again before braving that whole cycle again. Sounds fun, huh?

On the north side of this two-sided mountain, the upper lifts were T-bars because it was colder on that side and a chairlift up in the air was considered more dangerous on bitter cold days. Riding T-bars up steep slopes is about as hard as skiing down them when you are still an intermediate or lower-skilled skier. My heart often jumped up into my throat as my spot in line moved to the front. I then had to scurry to my spot next to my partner and get ready to grab the bar from the attendant, quickly place the bar under my rump, and lean back before the cable grabbed hold and yanked. Sometimes a yank on two lightweight people launched them in the air and they could only hope they landed with their skis still pointing straight up the hill. This T-bar would become somewhat of a nemesis years later when I approached it as a new amputee with outriggers.

The last year I skied on two legs was the year the safety brake on one of the double chairs broke. Normally, since a chairlift is heavily loaded all on one side, a very strong brake is employed if the lift has to stop for any reason to contend with the huge weight imbalance. If that brake fails, as it did that day, the lift can get going backwards very fast and whip people around the wheel at the bottom. This can cause horrible injuries. We could tell right away the brake had failed, but luckily our chair was not very high off the ground. We knocked off our skis and jumped into nice soft snow. Others did not have the presence of mind to do that or couldn't due to their elevation. Some people's backs broke as they whipped around at the bottom. It was the nightmare anyone who has ever ridden a chairlift has had. For days after, as they tried to fix that brake, they kept the chairs heavily loaded with sandbags for testing. We avoided that chair the rest of that week, even after they certified it as fixed.

Everyone in the family was required to take a solid week of full day lessons each year we went to Tremblant. This was part of the plan and no one questioned it. Morning and afternoon, everyone was in a class according to their skiing level. Full week lessons were a great way to improve our skiing. In an almost uncannily prescient way, one day my instructor directed our class to do one-legged skiing as a training drill. That morning we left our right ski and ski boot behind and wore a regular snow boot instead. We tucked our right foot behind the one on the ski. After lunch, we switched. It was hard to balance, and it was tremendously tiring. Furthermore, our skiing skills were not yet good enough to pull it off. But the following year, as a sixteen-year-old lying in a hospital bed looking down at a stump where my right leg had been, remembering that I had indeed skied on one ski was my one positive, shining light of hope.

My mother didn't choose the aggressive surgical front lines of medicine that her husband had. She chose pathology, a much more intellectual and cerebral branch of medicine, largely because it allowed saner hours that would enable her to have a family. Women physicians were still rare in her day and she was used to being surrounded by male physicians with all their bluster and testosterone. It helped a lot that she was six feet tall and looked them all in the eyes. She was not imposing, just quietly confident. She learned how to get her way without making the men around her feel like they had lost. When I became aware that almost every group in which she participated was all male, I asked her how it made her feel. She turned to me and said, "I never even noticed I was the only woman."

At home Mom was the most organized person I ever knew. It all started with breakfast. To keep herself organized, she assigned set breakfasts to days of the week. She never deviated. On any given day, breakfast choices were like Henry Ford's options on the Model T. On Monday you could have any thing you wanted, as long as it was cereal. You could have hot cereal in the winter, but Monday was cereal day one way or the other. Tuesday was soft-boiled egg day. Wednesday, French toast day. Thursday, scrambled eggs. Friday, pancakes. Saturday was help yourself. And Sunday was bacon and eggs day. It was cast in stone and never changed for the eighteen years I lived at home. It continued unabated into my mother's retirement. Naturally, I have never considered not following Mom's breakfast schedule throughout my life.

Dad had rules for everything. We were not allowed to wear blue jeans to school, so we all wore nice slacks to breakfast and then changed into jeans as soon as he left for work. We were not allowed to go around the house without shoes on. Dinners were regimented and formal. We sat at a big formal dining room table. We had intellectual exercises during dinner. We would have math tests, vocabulary quizzes, history games, and word puzzles. If you didn't know something it was thought you should know, you were embarrassed and motivated to learn so you could avoid being humiliated the next time. It created an extreme level of competition between the older kids because if you could get someone else to answer wrong, that person got the heat and you were off the hook. Despite how much I hated it, my father's approach toughened me up, emotionally and intellectually, in what would prove to be very important ways.

In the end, this was all pretty normal stuff.

When we are pushed hard and life throws us a major curve ball, what determines if we fight back and overcome or withdraw and give up? Is there something special, different, and rare in someone's personality—the core of how they operate and behave—that sets one person up to recover, get past normal, and even achieve supernormal?

I believe all human beings have phenomenal resilience when they are tested and allow themselves to exhibit that resilience. There is no middle ground in the face of extreme adversity. Either one caves and becomes a victim, or one totally compensates—perhaps even overcompensates—and comes out better, stronger, happier. The compensation against some sort of physical disability carries over to other aspects of life. Doctors knew this and documented it with polio survivors. Most polio survivors developed a "special relation to their bodies unknown to able-bodied persons. They experienced a new mastery over their muscles and movements, an element of control . . . that carried over into other aspects of their lives and probably accounts for why so many . . . excelled at school and work."[*]

No one I had known as a kid had been disabled or had dealt

---

[*] Lauro Halstead, "Post-Polio Syndrome," *Scientific American,* April 1998.

with serious adversity. Dad's parents had escaped Russia at the time of the pogroms, and much of our extended family who lived in Europe had been victims of the Holocaust. That was ancient history to which I had not been exposed. My dad had been, however, and he was subconsciously passing that on to me. Perhaps I had just enough experiences like the broken leg and dealing with a tough disciplinarian parent, and perhaps I had just enough of a willful personality to prepare me for what was to come. Or is it that, like the highly-studied polio survivors, there is a Survivor Syndrome that drives all humans faced with serious adversity to achieve and overachieve?

I believe, in the end, this discussion about being normal is really about ability versus disability. "Perhaps there is too much emphasis on disability rather than ability. . . . How many people actually know what their abilities are?" asks Jane Smith in *Trying to be Normal*. This is a great question. I believe people faced with a disability or some kind of disadvantage—think of the sightless person whose sense of hearing magnifies—test their abilities more than others and push past what seems like limitations. The most gratifying moment in the recovery and rehabilitation of a person inflicted by a disability is when someone able-bodied says they cannot compete with that person. It feels like you have arrived. The confidence it instills spreads throughout your personality and everything you do, giving you courage, fortitude, and happiness. This is the ultimate goal I wish for everyone faced with a disability, a personal crisis, or any life challenge. Fight back. Find a way to win even with something small. Find a small victory and build on it. Build and build to the point where you have found a place to excel beyond those who are not disabled. Suddenly you are there—back on a level playing field. Strong and happy.

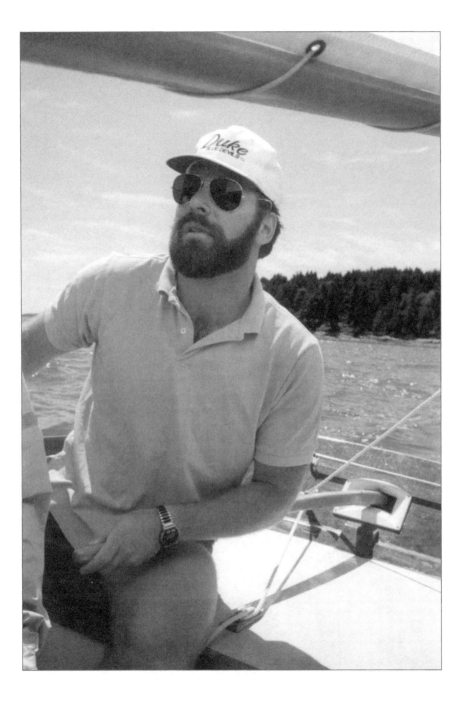

Part II—Ventures and Adventures

ven•ture |ˈven ch ər|[**]
noun. **1.** A risky or daring journey or undertaking. **2.** A business enterprise involving considerable risk.

ad•ven•ture |adˈven ch ər; əd-|
noun. **1.** An unusual and exciting, typically hazardous, experience or activity. **2.** A daring and exciting activity calling for enterprise and enthusiasm.

** Apple's OS X Dictionary

SIX

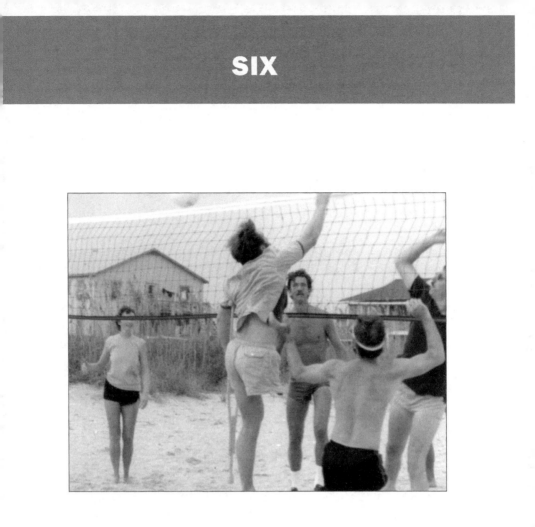

LEARNING TO LIVE

In three words I can sum up everything I've learned about life: It goes on.

— Robert Frost, poet

Nothing builds self-esteem and self-confidence like accomplishment.

— Thomas Carlyle, essayist

Self-esteem isn't everything; it's just that there's nothing without it.

— Gloria Steinem, feminist and journalist

Back from ski bumming and two quick quarters on campus, I was headed off on foreign study. I enrolled at the University of Strasbourg in Alsace, on the far eastern edge of France. Alsace had been a ping pong ball of annexation through history as it bounced back and forth between Germany and France. Strasbourg seemed to have retained the best of both. People had a strong work ethic, and the local beers were of highest German quality, but all the food and wine were of wonderful French quality.

The other Kalamazoo students on foreign study were juniors and I, being a senior, didn't know any of them. With no strong friendships to influence me, I felt freer with my choices of where to stay. Many students arranged to live in dorms, where they would surely all speak English to each other, but I chose to stay with a French family, the Éberlés. They spoke no English, even though Dr. Éberlé was an educated physician and his two boys were heading to medical school. I had taken three years of French, but I had not worked hard at it, and now I wished my language skills were better. I was no natural at learning a language, but I could get by. I was not afraid to blurt out what I thought was the right way to say something, which made the French want to help more than had I not tried.

During my introductory dinner, the Éberlés informed me that my bath day would be Wednesday. I was sure I must have misunderstood their French, but no, I had understood perfectly. They wanted me to fit into the culture, and apparently part of that was to smell bad. So I could bathe on Wednesdays. Only on Wednesdays. This was a well-to-do family, so it was not about the money; it was just culturally how it was done. Luckily, some of the other students were in the dorm, so I could go over there and shower on non-Wednesdays.

I loved being immersed in a different culture, but interesting surprises came along with it. My first dessert with my host family—on the same day I learned about my assigned bath day—was lemon pie. I love lemon pie. So I asked for and got a nice big piece. When I took my normal, large first bite, I found that I was chewing on slices of lemon rind. They never asked me, "Do you like rind with your lemon pie?" It was the second of many lessons I would have about different cultures.

My Ford Maverick had had enough at one hundred thousand miles. This was a great time and place to get a new car. Kalamazoo agreed that it was going to make getting around for me a heck of a lot easier—frankly, possible—and so they made an exception to the no-car-on-foreign-study rule. I arranged to get a US-legal VW Dasher (called a Passat in Europe, and later in the States) and picked it up at the factory in Stuttgart. My first weekend in Europe, I had to learn the train system and get myself to Stuttgart. Right away, I got to experience the autobahn and the crazy speeds at which Germans drive. Big, black Mercedes flew down the left lane at one hundred miles per hour or more with their left blinker constantly flashing. That meant get the heck out of the way and don't make them touch the brakes. It was hard not to get in their way though because, even with diligent mirror checking, pulling out to pass a truck that is only going seventy often resulted in one of those black monsters slamming on its brakes to slow to a piddling eighty-five or ninety. I ignored the rule of thumb that says don't push a new car really hard until it's broken in. I drove ninety-five on the autobahn right away. It was that or get creamed from behind. It's a very different driving culture in Germany, where even cops drive hot Porsches.

When I got my new car back to Strasbourg, my first task was to make my new Dasher left-footed. A garage, where no one spoke English, did the work by completely rerouting the accelerator linkage through the engine block wall back under the steering wheel to a relocated accelerator placed to the left of the brake. This made room for Herbie's foot to rest to the right of the brake, interfering with nothing. It worked great for me, but loaning the car to two-leggers created great consternation on their part. When faced with a peddle to the left of the brake, a two-legger's instinct is that it must be a clutch, which must always be pushed all the way down when starting from a standing stop. Several two-leggers bounced the Dasher off a number of curbs and drove through bushes before they learned it wasn't a clutch after all.

Because I was frequently over at the dorms to maintain a decent level of personal hygiene, I formed new friendships with some of the Kalamazoo juniors in my foreign study group. I frequently joined my new friends for meals. The cafeteria's only entrance was from the dorm parking lot, down a set of stairs through double doors, where it then wound through what looked like cattle pens to the stairs and up to where the food was served. The double doors were opened at precisely 6 p.m. Hungry students congregated on the stairs and in the parking lot quite a while before opening time. Anticipating opening time, the crowd would surge toward the doors, aided by gravity, pushing everyone down the stairs. Every night, girls at the front of the line were violently smashed up against the double doors or the sidewalls of the staircase, screaming in pain. The fact that the doors opened outward made the situation even more danger-ous. I couldn't stand seeing this. Since many of the screaming girls were our girls, I decided we needed to take matters into our own hands because the cafeteria workers would do nothing to help. For a few nights, long before the 6 p.m. opening, the largest guys in our group formed a human barrier across the top of the stairs. We placed our girls down at the bottom of the stairs, protected by us and with lots of space behind us in which they could roam. As opening time approached, the crowd couldn't stand to see this gap, and so they would start to push down the stairs toward the beckon-ing doors. But our barrier was made of large and strong boys, and we were determined not to let that happen anymore. It worked, but it was not particularly nice or safe, and it did not improve the French impression of Americans. It was a hugely positive experi-ence for me, however. I may have had a disability, but at six feet two inches I was one of the biggest guys, and I was stronger and bolder than the French or African students pushing and shoving, so I was able to join the other large boys in our group to help prevent the girls from getting squeezed.

Something strange and wonderful was happening. This was a long way from how things had felt just a few years earlier when I had been lying in a hospital bed wondering what, if anything,

I would be able to do physically ever again. Who would have believed back then that I'd ever be able to use the "er" suffix on words like *stronger* and *bolder*? I reveled in this newfound equality. Rebuilding my confidence after near total annihilation was a long, slow process. But it was happening. Like trust, confidence takes a long time to build up and a split second to eradicate. I wanted to push farther into this new territory, where I was not only on equal footing—so to speak—as two-leggers, but where I exceeded what many of them could do. It felt like a drug and I wanted more of it.

Having a car on foreign study was totally liberating. I took a road trip every weekend. The others in the group loved having me there with a car. My Dasher was like having a Golden Retriever puppy on a walk on the beach: everyone wants to be your friend. We took wine tours in the fall, tasting freshly-bottled Beaujolais Nouveau wine. The little towns we passed through had both sides of their already narrow roads packed with parked cars, while people tasted that village's offering before moving on to the next town to do it again. Barely a car width was left in which to drive between the parked cars.

The car was great for getting around Strasbourg, as walking to and from buses would have added a lot of wear and tear on my prosthetic skin-plastic interface. That skin-plastic interface, where the hard socket of the leg was held on to my five-inch stump with suction, was a constant source of problems. It hurt a lot. The friction often abraded and broke down the skin, sometimes resulting in bleeding. And if I perspired too much, I lost suction and the leg fell off, so I always had a safety belt to prevent that embarrassment. At the very least, it was a constant reminder that all was not normal. At the very worst, it made me feel downright crippled. The range of emotions an amputee, or any disabled person, can quickly go through is large. One moment I'd be skiing down High Rustler hearing admiring comments and the next my prosthesis knee would buckle and I'd fall flat on my face.

Before I left for France, my friend Geoff—the one who invited me to be sick in a bowl at his apartment during my chemotherapy treatments—who was a big Francophile and adored great French food, had challenged me to go to a famous Michelin three-star restaurant that, on his various gastronomic tours through France, he had missed. It was called Illhausen after the town of the same name in which it was located. That was just a bit south of Strasbourg, but it was way out of the way of Geoff's most recent tour of the *Cote d'Azure*. My assignment was to find someone to go with, make reservations, have a great meal, and record every minute detail of the experience so Geoff could feel as though he had actually gone there himself. In return, he would pay for the whole affair.

I chose Betty LeGal—the stunningly beautiful daughter of a former colleague of Mom's who happened to live in Strasbourg—to be my companion on my adventure. Job one then was to ask Betty to go with me. Illhausen was well known locally as an out-of-reach, only-for-the-rich restaurant, and so she was thrilled by my invitation. I called for a reservation in October and the first opening for a table for two was a Sunday in December, and only for lunch. I took what I could get. When the day of our reservation arrived, I drove with Betty down to the tiny town of Illhausen and found the restaurant. It was an old brick building right on the river that runs through town. The inside was nicely remodeled, and the wall facing the river had been completely replaced with glass, giving patrons the sense of hanging in midair, suspended over the quiet, fog-enshrouded river, as they dined. My first observation was that we were the only people under sixty in the place. The other was that *objets d'art* on the wall looked very expensive. Suddenly I worried if the mechanics of my knee might suddenly fail and I would stumble right toward a wall and take out thousands of dollars worth of art. The thick, white pile carpet actually made this scenario more likely. I prudently moved to the center of the hallway and stayed completely away from the walls.

Four waiters were assigned to just the two of us. The first stood behind me, and every time one of us took a sip of wine, he replenished exactly that one sip in our glasses, returning then to his stoic palace guard pose. The second just handled appetizers like the *pâté de fois gras*. This was served in a crock dish that was placed on a bed of ice that, in turn, sat on a silver platter. Next to this was a pitcher of very hot water in which were placed two silver spoons. On our plates were three triangular pieces of thin toast. The appetizer waiter took out the first hot, silver spoon and laid it gently on the surface of the pâté, which he spun in its crock dish sitting on its bed of ice. While it was spinning, he lifted, with his hot spoon, a thin slice of pâté of perfect thickness, which, with a flick of his wrist, he deposited perfectly on the first piece of toast. He then switched to the other spoon, always using a reheated one for each sliver of pâté. The third waiter was our entrée waiter, who focused on our main meal. The fourth one served only our desserts.

Betty—being a woman—had a menu that had no prices; mine did. I felt very intimidated and could swear that all the over-sixties were staring at us wondering what the heck we were doing in their restaurant. It was hard to enjoy the meal. Even drinking wine was stressful with the humorless palace guard right behind me refilling our glasses after every sip.

We made it through the meal and out the door without incident. No faux pas that I knew of and no crashes into any expensive objects. I wrote a multi-page detailed account of my afternoon at Illhausen for Geoff, and he quite happily made good on his payment promise.

The university classes were large, with hundreds of both French and African students sitting on long wooden benches in the tightly packed lecture halls. By design, we foreign study students took no classes in our major. I took French History, French Civilization, French Art, and French Language. No math. All classes were taught in French. I did not take classes very seriously. None of us did. I was there to soak up the culture while I could. My idea of study abroad was to immerse myself in my chosen country, and immerse was what I was going to do.

I was starting to write postcards to and think a lot about Carole, who had recently split up with her husband. The cool thing was that she was writing back. For the first time I began to feel like maybe I had a chance with her.

Many nights when we were not fighting off hoards at the cafeteria and I was not getting a nice meal with my host family or Betty's family, we learned to love a classic, cheap French meal. We'd get a baguette, a bottle of Beaujolais wine, and a hunk of Port Salut cheese. The entire meal might cost $4, less than the cost of a gallon of gas in France.

Occasionally, I was invited to a French student party. An American student visiting one of those parties always got the royal treatment. They asked what music I liked. I created quite a ruckus when I stumbled into a very embarrassing colloquialism by asking for "ZZ Top." The letter *Z* is pronounced "zed" in French. When pronounced as it is in American English, "Z Z" is the French child's word for penis. So, using a child's slang, I had asked them to play "Penis Top." The entire party laughed so hard no one could tell me what stupid thing I had said. I just sat there taking it in, looking confused and clueless. Eventually someone explained the slang and we then went on to listen to some "Zed Zed Top."

The two Éberlé brothers, Michel and Paul, were both headed for medical school. They were diehard skiers, too, and invited me to join them at their place at the Flaine ski resort near Geneva. It was great to be skiing a big mountain again, and they were very good skiers. We had fun tearing up that mountain, tearing being the operative word. My worst skiing crash ever involving me and another person occurred on that trip.

Michel and Paul said we had to get from the small hill we were on, across a large flat area, all the way to the other side to a lift. To make it and avoid a long walk, we had to schuss straight down in a tuck from our current perch all the way across that huge, flat snow-field. The only problem was that ahead of us were two older people snowplowing back and forth, taking up the whole slope. We would each have to carefully time our run so that we went right between the two of them when they were both on the apogee of their orbits. It worked fine for Paul, and then for Michel too. Initially, I seemed to have it timed right in turn, but just as I neared the couple, they both decided to change their rhythm by doing one quick turn, at which point they were headed straight back toward each other and right into my path. I had time neither to turn nor to stop. All I could do was hunker down and brace myself for impact. After the crash, the slope looked like a yard sale. My equipment, their equipment, our hats, our goggles, everything was spread all over the place. Then the swearing started. In French, of course. They were livid. And I was sorry, as it clearly was my fault, they were elderly and I could have hurt them badly. But I could not be sorry enough for them, apologizing in my weak French. All I could do was try to look sorry as I picked up all my stuff and headed down to where Paul and Michel were waiting. My punishment was that I had to push myself using outriggers across that large, flat field, since I no longer had nearly enough speed to get across it using my previous momentum.

It had now been two years since metastases of the cancer had taken my lung and given me the death sentence, and I was still going strong. Better than strong. I was thriving and picking up the pace; something kept making me want to live hard and fast and get it all in while I could. Not having any other great idea about what to do next when I got home from France, and since I was a senior and had to figure this out while still on foreign study, I decided then and there to go to graduate school. Another inauspicious decision-making process: *I'm not dead yet and I can't think of anything better to do, so maybe I'll go to graduate school.* I knew I did not want to go into medicine. Not only were both my parents physicians, but my older brother had gone that route as well. Not for me. I had headed down a different path early on. I liked math a lot. And during countless dinners as children, when both parents dominated the dinner table conversation with discussion of "cases" and of people with tumors and gangrene, I was actually repelled by the idea of it as a career. Furthermore, the idea of getting a job at all didn't make sense to me right now because I was still doubtful I would be around much longer. I liked school and I liked math, so continuing with both of those things was the best option I could come up with. Not the most inspiring rationale for getting a master's degree in math, but it was all I had.

The only place within several hundred miles of Strasbourg to take the required Graduate Record Exam was at a US Army base in Ramstein, Germany. I signed up and drove to the small town near the base and stayed at a rustic, little German hotel. Naturally, the people taking the exam were ninety-nine percent American service men and women. No one else from my foreign study group would be taking it, as they were all juniors. Afterward, I felt like I had done well on the exam.

My time in France went very fast. Two quarters were over just like that and it was back to Kalamazoo. My modified plan left me one more quarter of my senior year, and I would graduate in the spring, miraculously on time.

I found out Carole's divorce was nearly official, and the day it became final, I asked her out for our first date. She accepted and

I took her to one of the lousiest movies either of us has ever seen. It didn't matter. She seemed to like me and that felt really good. I was determined to take it slow and not blow it. Since this was just our first date, I gave her only a peck on the cheek; I would build on that very carefully. Besides, I was very inexperienced in matters of romance and relationship and I was scared to take that big, fateful step with her.

We had three dates. Then we had a fourth. I was twenty-one and I was having a real relationship with a woman for the first time in my life. And it was with the woman I would eventually marry. It was a miracle that I'd lived long enough to experience sex. I was really smitten by Carole. The fact that she liked me and was not at all bothered by my missing a leg was incredibly attractive to me.

During that spring of my senior year, Carole came up to school. I took her to a park that had a big hill with a view. I thought it was a romantic spot for Kalamazoo. We climbed the hill and I made a big speech about what she meant to me and how this was the big one for me. Maybe a little of the female caregiver instinct was coming out, or maybe something about my drive and determination intrigued her. Or perhaps she thought, *What do I have to lose; this might be fun*. Regardless, to my delight she was willing to play it out and see what happened.

That summer after graduation I had two jobs, both in hospital labs. One was back at the same old vascular surgery lab where Carole and Nellie worked, and the other was at the hospital where my mother worked. I stayed with Carole and her three-year-old son Brendan two nights a week.

As all of this progressed with Carole, I was faced with a real dilemma. I had applied and gotten into Northwestern University's masters in mathematics program. My plan was to keep learning and doing as much other fun stuff as possible until the other shoe (and I) dropped. But it hadn't dropped yet, and now here I was with Carole and Brendan. She had just been accepted to the Physician Assistant program at Duke University. At this early stage in my very first real relationship, if I went to Evanston, Illinois, and she went to Durham, North Carolina, I knew our relationship had no chance. I had to very quickly figure out how I, too, could become a Blue Devil.

I wanted to switch from Northwestern to Duke, but Duke said it was too late for me to apply for their graduate program. I would probably not be accepted this late, they told me, and there was no way I would get any stipend to defray my tuition costs. They said I was free to apply anyway, so I did—to the Biomedical Engineering PhD program.

I got a fast response: not only would they accept me into the PhD program in biomedical engineering, but they would also give me a full stipend. This was thanks to the caliber of Kalamazoo, good grades, and a very strong GRE score from that test I had taken on the army base in Germany. I walked away from a non-refundable deposit at Northwestern, never looking back, and entered Duke's PhD program. Biomedical Engineering seemed as good as anything. Roger, the head of the lab where Carole and I had met, was a biomedical engineer. I liked the way he applied an engineering discipline to a biological science. Besides, from my limited exposure to them, I liked computers and saw a great application for them in medicine. What went through my mind was, *Well, I am still alive against all odds. Carole seems great. A PhD is a challenge most people cannot meet. So I'll be with Carole and attack that PhD challenge with gusto.*

Clean breaks with vestiges of the past are a nice way to symbolically mark major life transitions. For me, it was helpful to make these clean breaks dramatic. It seemed so far like each of my major life transitions—from amputation during high school heading off to college, and from metastatic cancer, surgery, and chemotherapy during college heading off to a relationship and graduate school—represented an equally dramatic break from a pretty horrible set of experiences. I decided this would be a good time to dramatically liberate myself from the cane. I had now been using it for over three years. I no longer really needed it physically, but I did psychologically. It had at many times been quite a nuisance, such as when I needed two hands to carry things. And I had not always used it as just an assistive device—at best not the way an assistive cane is supposed to be used. When my football-playing roommate was with me in our dorm room, he considered me a formidable roughhousing opponent just because of my upper body strength. He felt like I had the upper hand in arm wrestling matches that he felt, as a fine upstanding football player, he by all rights should be winning. So when we were out in the open walking around campus, he loved to rush up from nowhere and get a quick jab in on me, then quickly flee to a safe distance away that I could not cover nearly as quickly as he could. But one day I realized my cane could indeed cover that distance easily. I let fly after one particularly sharp jab he gave my arm. My aim was good. The cane clipped him on the back of a leg and he went down in a heap. Not really hurt, we both started laughing. And counter to what logic would dictate, it was he who felt guilty for the cane now being broken and he ran off to find strong duct tape to fix it.

My clean break from the cane, as the representation of all the dependence I had had on others and on the fear I had had to manage ever since the death threat, came at the same time as college graduation. With Carole and me planning to move to Durham for graduate school, I made a big proclamation.

"I will no longer be needing a cane," I said, thrusting my trusty old wooden companion, still held together with my roommate's duct tape, into the back of a closet. Since then it has only come out to be loaned to family and friends who have knee replacements or other temporary leg disabilities. For me, it's a reminder of the past and no more useful than one's freshman year textbooks.

We went down to Durham to look for places to live. Carole was adamant that it was too early and it would put too much pressure on our relationship for us to move in together. That was before she got the sticker shock of rent times two. We decided to move in together because we couldn't afford not to. Like my criteria for finishing college after the ski bum season, my graduate school decision was based on "because I can't think of anything better to do." In the same vein, our living together and taking the relationship to the next level was based on "because we can't afford to live separately." An inauspicious beginning to be sure, but sometimes miracles do happen.

We had to be in Durham for the beginning of school in August, but our townhouse would not be available for about a week. Along with Brendan, we had to live in a tent in a state park in the ninety-five-degree, late-August heat of North Carolina. My main job was to swipe the sweat bees and mosquitoes off Carole after dinner, while she tried to study at the campsite picnic table by the light of our bonfire. I also had to keep a three-year-old reasonably happy and quiet. Brendan was a challenge, partly, we found out much later, because he had Attention-Deficit Disorder (ADD). ADD didn't allow him to focus on one thing, and it interfered with his impulse control. He was also a challenge for me because I was twenty-one and suddenly and unexpectedly a stepfather to a three-year-old.

At the outset, my new biomedical engineering department jumped to the conclusion that, since I had an artificial leg and since one of their faculty's research specialized in leg prosthetics, I would want to make that my research area. They further concluded that I would want to be a guinea pig on his prosthetic projects. All of this without so much as asking me.

In fact, I had no interest in making prosthetics my research area. I was still quite uncomfortable being around other amputees. I didn't want to make being an amputee a club activity nor a focus in my life any more than it had to be. I didn't think of myself as disabled, and when I was around other people who had lost limbs, I could not stand how some of them just whined. The most ridiculous conversations I heard at one group I attended began with, "So which is worse to lose, a leg or an arm?"

I did agree to be a guinea pig because I had a strong desire to see prosthetic devices improved and to have it get easier for first-timers to learn how to use them. I recalled that it had taken me at least six months to learn how to walk with the prosthesis unassisted by crutches. This was too long and something needed to be done to shorten and improve that process. This was precisely the goal of the first project in which they wanted me to participate.

The research idea was to help the brain relearn how to walk with a new and more powerful sensory input. At the time, visual senses were all an amputee had to help him understand the position of his foot and knee. He couldn't tell where the mechanical knee and foot were by any sense of feel. All he could do was look down and see that his foot was safely out in front of him and that his knee was straight and locked, meaning it was safe to put weight on it. If it was not straight and locked—like if the foot got caught under a rug or had come down on a marble—he'd fall. With no proprioceptors feeding knee position back to the brain, amputees use vision to tell their brain if the leg is properly positioned. Not being able to feel through the prosthetic knee what position the leg is in, or feel the foot when it hits the ground, makes learning how to walk on a prosthesis difficult.

Sound was the new sensory input they wanted to add. Sound would be used to provide strong, repeated feedback about where the foot was, thereby freeing up the amputee's eyes to focus elsewhere, not constantly down at their knee and foot. The scheme provided for sensors in the prosthetic toe and heel connected to a transducer, which in turn was connected to a hearing aid. The wearer would hear a click and a tone at one frequency when the heel hit the ground, and a different frequency tone and corresponding click when the toe left the ground. With every step he would hear click-da-da-da-da-dee-dee-dee-click in his ear. Others could hear it, too. It was annoying, but the idea seemed to make sense. A huge issue was that the research team did not hook up all this fancy sensory feedback stuff to the leg and knee I knew. They didn't use Herbie. Instead, they used the very cheapest available knee. I started click-da-da-dee-dee-clicking all over the place: up and down the halls of the biomedical engineering department; on the treadmill in a controlled environment; to and from my car; around my townhouse. Click-da-da-dee-dee-click all the time.

The professor in charge of this project was the same guy who worked as an expert witness against aqua slide manufacturers and on behalf of ski resorts regarding head and neck injuries. He came up with the designs for motorcycle and football helmets by dropping orangutan cadavers down elevator shafts in Duke buildings and studying the way their skulls and brain tissue were affected by the impact.

Biomedical engineering graduate students who received a stipend were required to take the normal four courses and then work as a teaching assistant or lab assistant in a fifth course in an unfamiliar area. This was essentially a tricky way to get us to take a fifth course. For me that course was an introductory electronics lab. Building stereos and TVs from kits did not teach me about the theory, much less the practical implementation of how circuits work. I knew how to read color codes on resistors, but that was all.

This was all totally new material to me, making me way behind my students.

One day we had a lab in the class and the students were tasked with building circuits that featured different-sized resistors. Resistors are little ceramic tubes with wires coming out of each end, and the ceramic has color-coded lines painted on it to identify its size.

I was carrying a metal box with about five hundred thousand resistors, all neatly organized according to the color codes and slotted into hundreds of little compartments for each size. Of course, I was also click-da-da-dee-dee-clicking as I came down the hall carrying this large, heavy, metal box. Just as I came into the room where all the nice, fresh-faced undergraduates were patiently waiting for their allotment of resistors delivered by their friendly T.A., the cost-saving knee they used on the guinea pig leg buckled backwards and collapsed catastrophically. I went flying, but more importantly, the heavy metal box went flying, too. Corner of the resistor box met corner of the nearby lab table. As we know, gravity works fast, and that box hit the table hard. The impact caused most of the five hundred thousand resistors to explode out of the box and to spread out over the stunned students in a beautiful fan-shaped pattern of randomly color-coded little missiles. The sharp corner of the box also got one more shot at me: it sliced open my forearm.

So there I was on the floor, arm bleeding and with a non-functional leg. The floor was covered with thousands and thousands of resistors. I quickly regained a modicum of composure and told the students that the purpose of today's lab was to learn how to color code resistors, and that we would do that by picking up resistors from their random placement across the floor and putting them back into the box in their correct slots, calling out their correct resistance value as we went.

That afternoon, I ceremoniously returned the now broken cheap leg, with its sensors, tone generators, and hearing aid, and resigned from the study and from a relationship with professor McElheney as my advisor. I would find a research project and advisor in something that really interested me and that did not threaten more bodily injury.

Medical computing seemed like a much better fit for me. It tied back to what I had been doing at the hospital lab in Detroit. It was one of the strengths of the Duke department. Best of all, it had nothing to do with prosthetics, aqua slides, Orangutan cadavers, or hearing aids.

It was 1978, very early in the life of UNIX, the ancestor of Linux, MacOS X, and much of the work since in computer operating systems. Recently out of Bell Labs, it had been offered to a handful of universities, including Duke. Bob was my new advisor, so my new home was in the basement of the student health building where he had his offices and labs. I was given a Digital Equipment Corporation PDP-11/40 mini computer running UNIX to administer. This was another died-and-gone-to-heaven moment for me. I had an office of my own with large windows right in front of my new charge. The twenty-megabyte disk for this machine was bigger than a washing machine, yet it held only a thousandth of what a small iPod holds today. An array of lights tracked what was going in and out of that disk drive. I got so familiar with those blinking light patterns that I could tell what the machine was doing just by watching the patterns from my desk. When the machine had to be taken down for maintenance or problem resolution, I toggled into a set of front panel switches a sequence of machine instructions (where switch on and switch off corresponded to ones and zeros) that created a booting program that brought up UNIX and readied the machine to run. The machine was part of a system used throughout the medical center for patient record maintenance.

I started to explore ideas for research, but mostly I played a lot. I took a lot of computer science classes and just the few required biomedical engineering core classes. I got in on the ground floor of computing as minicomputers took over from the mainframe generation. Bob's lab got lots of cool, new toys. I got my hands on the first PC using an Intel microprocessor. It was called an "Altair" and was programmed by inserting machine instructions through front panel switches. There was no UNIX to run; it was bare metal, as we liked to say. I had to write a program for anything I wanted this little computer to do. I wrote a program to read paper tapes and another one to interface to a Teletype machine. I wrote a little text editor and I played around with lots of little programs to do simple computations. I entered so many programs through those little pointy, front-panel switches that my fingertips got sore and bloodied.

Eventually, I came up with a project for my PhD with Bob. I had completed most of my coursework, so it was time to create and then meet with a full PhD committee to get their buy-in for my project. That meeting did not go as expected. They evaluated my proposal and said it was way too much computers and way too little medicine to be called Biomedical Engineering. That had to be adjusted, they declared, and to get me shifted over more to the medicine side of biomedicine, they now required that I take Medical School Physiology. I was stunned, and I was extremely disappointed with Bob for doing such a poor job preparing me for the meeting and preparing the committee for my proposal. But I took their rejection to heart and enrolled in the Med School Physiology class.

It was a huge class—all the first year Med School students took this course together. It was a formal lecture class with no professor interaction. Just get the big, fat book, go to class, take copious notes, memorize, and study for exams. It was exactly what I had assumed medical school was like. The problem was I didn't have the necessary biology background. Sure, I had taken a biology class in high school, as well as one chemistry class, but I knew more about biology from overhearing snippets of medical talk between my parents than from any class. I was one of those people who thought protein was simply something you got from steak. I was lost, and that was a new and terrifying feeling for me. I had never struggled in a class before. I went to the head instructor for help. He impatiently said to me, "This class is for medical students. You graduate students just fill in the cracks. I do not have time for you. Find a fellow student who will help you." In that moment, I snapped and decided I wanted out of Biomedical Engineering. I started to look into what it would take to switch to Computer Science. But I refused to fail and I would not quit a class even if I didn't really understand proteins. I ended up getting the first and only C in my life in "Physiology For Medical Students Not Graduate Students Who Just Fill In The Cracks."

By now I had taken many computer science classes. I loved learning about operating systems, especially getting to write one of my own. I loved numerical analysis where programs could be written to perform tasks like computing integrals from calculus and computing pi to umpteen digits. I was enthralled with the accuracy of computers and the limitations that they had and loved designing algorithms, the mathematical, problem-solving recipes that are the basis for how computers work. Computer science felt like a great fit, so I approached the chairman of the computer science department. He had hinted to me while he was teaching numerical analysis that I should really be a computer scientist, so I knew he would be receptive. He was thrilled to help me switch over. He would take care of everything; I just had to tell my current advisor, Bob.

Bob was livid. This was not going to happen to him, he said. In fact, he declared, "If you go through with this and leave me and the Department of Biomedical Engineering, I will see to it that you have to leave the entire university."

This was the biggest non-medical crisis that I had faced in my life so far. I fully believed he could and would make my life at Duke miserable, and that he did have the power to make me leave. Duke and University of North Carolina at Chapel Hill had thoroughly intertwined their computer science departments so they could offer a combined and much richer graduate experience. Certain courses each department required were offered only at the other school. I had already taken two courses at Chapel Hill, and I knew many of the professors and graduate students. I went to UNC to explore my options to enroll in their graduate program. It was not going to be a slam-dunk transfer, so I explored other graduate departments at UNC as well. At Duke, however, the chairman of computer science was vehement that Bob was not going to get away with this behavior. He did some amazing behind the scenes political maneuvering and came back to tell me that I was in. I was now a Duke Computer Science graduate student in good standing, and Bob was blocked from doing anything to stop me. Problem solved. No further issues with Bob ever occurred, but I still tried to avoid seeing him around campus.

I had lost a year and had to use that year to complete all the coursework requirements in my new department. I also had to use that year to formulate a new computer science PhD research project.

A buzz began to infiltrate the progressive computer science and electrical engineering departments like Duke, Carnegie-Mellon,

Berkeley, Stanford, and MIT. That buzz was called VLSI design. Very Large Scale Integration was about building microchips that could perform significant computations in something the size of a pencil eraser. Universities were teaching people how to design these chips, and they were getting access to fabrication facilities to build real hardware. Duke brought in a visiting faculty member named Neil Weste from Bell Labs who was going to get us on the forefront of this area. He was also going to help the Research Triangle Area realize the first fabrication facility of its own so that we could build all the chips the students and researchers needed.

I took the course. I saw VLSI as a fertile area for my research focus, and I got Neil to be my research advisor. My co-advisors were two very famous people in computer science from UNC named Fred Brooks and Henry Fuchs. Not only was Fred the creator of the IBM 360 operating system, he also wrote the most famous book in computer science about that experience, *The Mythical Man-Month*. Henry was also very well known and a respected member of a community of researchers focused on computer graphics. Much of the results of his work can be seen in movie animation, video games, and the graphics on computers, movie special effects, and TV.

As a computer science graduate student, I upgraded from Bob's PDP 11/40 to a PDP 11/70 computer, which was newer and had more than twice the capacity. Two other students and I joined up to become the Three Musketeers of Duke's graduate students. Durward Rogers was a graphics genius. Steve Daniel, who was just as smart and an incredible programmer, rounded out our trio. We did ground breaking work on computer graphics, VLSI design, the first Internet News reader program, a great early computer game called Colossal Cave Adventure, and many other minor projects. It was a fun time of exploration, learning, and teamwork.

Our shared computer science graduate student offices had standard-issue, university, linoleum floors, but the hallways in our building were carpeted. Lars Nyland was a graduate student who had the office right across the hall from ours. We often visited and collaborated with each other. His desk was just inside his office door. On the opposite wall from two side-by-side desks were several floor-to-ceiling, heavily book-laden bookcases. One day when I stopped by, I stood over the junction of the hallway carpet and the office floor linoleum. My prosthesis heel came down on the half-inch-wide metal junction between carpet and floor. Because the carpet side was higher, my heel had lots of pressure while the toe had none. That put a lot of torque on the knee and it "broke." That means that when it was supposed to be locked and hold me up, it reacted to the pressure almost as if it thought I was walking and gave way. Instinctively, I reached up for something to grab onto to keep from falling. That something was the full height bookcase just in front of Lars. It was not bolted to the wall. Now, in addition to a two-hundred-pound man coming down fast toward Lars, a fully-loaded bookcase capable of crushing both of us was, too. Lars had great instincts. He launched himself out of his chair toward the bookcase with enough force to reverse its momentum and probably save both our lives. It was a reminder of the fragile line I walked between being the robust man I was beginning to think I was and someone with a disability that would capriciously humiliate me. It's the demon anyone with a disability lives with constantly.

Carole was now a full-fledged Physician Assistant and working at a local clinic. It was beginning to seem like I really might be sticking around the world of the living. I wanted to grab hold of Carole and make a commitment. I wanted stability. I wanted normalcy. And I wanted Carole. I decided it was time to ask Carole to marry me. We had been living together now for four years. It was five years post cancer, and everyone, even insurance companies, said five years was magic and I could now relax and plan on living. The relax part was hard though.

We started to think about kids. We had Carole's six-year-old, Brendan, but I wanted my own kids, too. Having kids would be a beyond miraculous turnaround from a near-certain death, and that fact did not escape me. We were not going to have kids unless we were married. Carole knew that no one had ever survived what had happened to me. She knew there was still a significant risk, but she wanted to get married and have kids, too. This Midwestern Catholic girl actually was a risk-taker after all.

A cloud of fear and doubt does not lift easily. A significant part of that cloud is indelible and permanent. It had worked its way into lots of dark little nooks and crannies in my brain, my personality, my soul. Every year that goes by lessens it a little. But it will never vanish completely. There are too many constant reminders, and the ways that it worked its way into my personality are, to a large extent, permanent.

I was paranoid about having children. *Was it possible that my cancer was genetic? Did they know for sure it was not?* I did not want to take any chances. I wanted any genetic tests that existed and I wanted to talk and talk with experts until I became convinced that what had happened to me was not going to be passed on through my genes. Only then would I agree that having kids made sense. Even if cancer was not a genetic risk, I needed to know whether the chemotherapy had done any damage to my sperm that might result in unhealthy or deformed offspring. After all, I still very clearly remembered how caustic those chemicals were that had been coursing through my body killing lots of cells. All tests resulted in a green light for us to go ahead and have children.

Carole's Physician Assistant student group was very social. We formed friendships through that group that are our deepest life-long friendships. Susan and Eric were PAs who, along with their spouses, Pat and Cristin, respectively, became our closest friends. As the wedding plans formed up, never ones to be accused of being standard and traditional, Carole and I decided to honeymoon before the wedding. Moreover, we decided it would be more fun not to go alone, but to go with all of our best friends. This was the first of many vacations we would take as a group that included Susan, Pat, Eric, Cristin, and occasionally a few others.

This trip had the theme "prenuptial alert." Every trip thereafter would have a theme that we would typically beat to death throughout our vacation week. That was part of the fun of our group—our themes and the relentless beating of them over each other's heads. In this case, whenever I was seen (or heard) snuggling (or more) in any way with Carole, out came the cry, "prenuptial alert," from the closest member of the self-appointed *propriety enforcement committee*. This happened even when they heard something mildly suspicious through the walls of our bedroom. This first vacation set the tone for a wonderful lifetime of friendship and mutual support from this group, all tied together through the PA connection.

Our wedding was held in my parent's yard. My family wanted to host the wedding in their beautiful backyard that I had worked so hard to help construct. The brick patio I had built the last summer I was two-legged was holding up perfectly. The stone walkways I had painstakingly laid down were settled in, and the gardens all around had had time to grow and mature. Carole and I wanted to dress for the ceremony, but as fast as possible afterward, we wanted everyone to change into play clothes for a game of softball and maybe some volleyball. Oh, and then if there was time left over, we'd eat, drink, and dance.

The ceremony, held in the garden with its late-May flowers and vibrant green grass, was presided over by our dear friend, Pat, who was the Methodist minister of our wedding. He was marrying an ex-Catholic and a non-practicing Jew, so he promised to mention Christ the minimal required number of times.

The minute the ceremony was over, we took over the front yard and played many hours of softball. I was the pitcher for my team, pitching with my leg on. When I batted, I had pinch runners who took off from my right at the crack of the bat. I played volleyball with no leg and with one crutch. Although no one said a wedding followed by softball and volleyball was weird, I am sure they thought it.

We had already had the honeymoon before the wedding, so afterward we hustled back to Durham for Carole's job and my graduate work. I moved pretty fast on the dissertation, and at the four-year point I had a one-hundred-page document done. My main advisor had gone back to Bell Labs, but remained on my committee; I needed a different main advisor. His name was Arny Rosenberg. He was no relation, but certainly the source of lots of jokes, which I encouraged by calling him "Uncle Arny." In turn, I was his first-ever graduate student advisee. He was a pure theoretical computer scientist—almost a pure mathematician—so we were indeed strange bedfellows. We were thrown together because I liked and respected him a lot, as he did me. In addition, he was working on the VLSI problem from a theoretical standpoint, so a tenuous research connection existed between us. Besides, there were no better options. He felt the same way. He told me that I was a hard-nosed pragmatic son of a gun (he made that sound like an affliction) in a theoretical computer science department where no one ever proposed to build real software. We were like oil and water, but he thought association with a pragmatic systems builder would balance his being such a pure theoretician, so we both agreed to try to make it work.

He looked at my one-hundred-page document, confirmed I had done sufficient research, and proclaimed the document complete. I was ready to leap up and start high-fiving, but before I could, he went on to say that I was still a year away from being done. I couldn't believe what I was hearing. I thought I was done and had beaten every person's challenge that I could not possibly do this in four years after changing departments. Actually, getting a PhD at all—even in five years—was a challenge most people acknowledged was beyond them, so I was still achieving things most people thought I could not.

Arny said his issue with my work was communication skills. He considered great researchers who could not communicate to be failures. He felt I needed to write and speak more effectively before he would schedule my defense. His requirement was that I write two journal papers and give two conference presentations on my work, and then, and only then, would he schedule the dissertation defense.

Carole got pregnant and her due date was a huge motivation for me to finish. I didn't need such huge motivation, but now I had a date by which I had to be done. Unlike writing and research schedules, hers was very unlikely to slip. She wanted to take a significant amount of time off after the baby, which I strongly supported, so I needed to make up her lost salary. In the end, I cut it very close. I had to work like a dog. I stopped exercising, stopped working in the yard, and in fact stopped nearly everything not directly supporting getting my PhD finished. That worried Carole and one day she said to me, "Will you ever help around the yard again?" That hurt. But I knew I could not let up for fear of losing my focus on finishing.

I wrote the papers. I gave the talks. I updated the dissertation. I prepared for my defense. Anticipation of the defense was thoroughly intimidating, but the actual event was far different. Somehow, I managed to get two members of the committee arguing with each other for forty-five minutes. I sat very quietly while they went at each other. I wanted to disappear into the walls while they argued away, knowing that after a while, when they tired, they would probably have to pass me. The one defending my work was my advisor Arny, and he won so I won. Done. In spite of incredible odds, I had a PhD. I had finished in time. It was May 1983. Zachary was born at the end of June. I had indeed cut it close.

This was all pretty amazing. Not only had I defied the odds of survival, but I'd also gotten married. I had just gotten a PhD, which most people admitted they cannot or will not do, death threat notwithstanding. I was fighting back and winning. To top it all, I had a son. Every father is awed by fatherhood. More so for me perhaps because, by all rights, I should not have even been alive. A son was the ultimate visible affirmation of my survival.

We held an authentic North Carolina *pig picking* graduation party in the backyard of our home in Rougemont, North Carolina. I cooked half a pig in an old converted oil drum from 6 a.m. to 8 p.m. Normal people hire someone to do this, but not me. No, I had to do it the hard way. I rented the oil drum cooker and bought the cleaned and prepared pig. At dawn the day of the party, I got the coals started and then, for the next fourteen hours, I tended that fire constantly. By the end of the day, I had singed my eyebrows and embedded grease in every pore of my body. The quartered pig was pinned between two pieces of fencing and placed over warm, but not overly hot, coals. Slow cooking is critically important. The pig had to be turned often, and the entire fencing contraption had to be flipped. I ended up with the greasy pig right up against my chest. The coals had to be tended constantly to keep them warm but not too hot. The pig was scheduled—as were everyone's hunger pangs—for 6 p.m. By the time it was finally done at 8, some people were desperate and pretty unhappy, but tolerant. I don't remember the party much because I was not really at it. I was at the pig cooker.

My first job was to be part of the founding team at the Microelectronics Center of North Carolina. At twenty-six, I was anointed vice president. To show how proud I was, I started wearing suspenders. Carole's loss of salary was exactly the difference between my Duke stipend and my new MCNC salary of $45,000. Durward and Steve, the other two-thirds of our graduate student three musketeers—Porthos and Aramis to my Atho—came to join my new team while continuing to work on their degrees. Duke was part owner of MCNC; each member of the MCNC team, including me, had adjunct appointments at the university, so naturally we had lots of students flowing in and out.

My new MCNC team's mission was to turn my PhD research into a commercial product. Make no mistake; I was not a "real" VP, as I was still hacking away on code. I just went to a bunch of meetings in my suspenders and felt important. My colleagues at the VP level were semi-retired, very experienced, famous people in their fields. I was still wet behind the ears, but thought I knew a lot. I must have been unbearably annoying to them.

We decided that my cells that survived the chemotherapy had overcompensated and gotten very strong. My hair had grown back coarser, and it turns out that I'm the last of the boys in the family to lose it. Some other important cells must have also become resilient because before even really trying for another kid, Carole got pregnant again.

In spite of being a medical person, Carole took the risk of no birth control while she was still breastfeeding, knowing we planned to have another baby some time soon. She did indeed get pregnant much sooner than we had planned. Zac and Joanna are not technically the thirteen months apart to qualify as "Irish twins," but with only a sixteen-month gap between them, we got some of the same effects, both good and not so good. Joanna coming so fast meant Carole had to stop breastfeeding poor little Zac much sooner than she (or he) wanted. We joke that he never completely forgave Joanna or us for that insult. Because of medical technology, we knew she was Joanna quite far in advance so we could call her by name in utero. Because Zac was delivered caesarian, Carole had to have Joanna that way as well; therefore, we could plan in advance not only her name, but also the date and time of her birth.

Normally when I was finished with work I was also done with my leg for the day. Wearing it is uncomfortable, and it's a constant battle to keep the skin that rubs against plastic from breaking down. With two babies and only two adults in the house, I had to learn how to carry a kid while on crutches. Carrying little babies like that up and down stairs was a challenge. I used one hand to hold the baby close to my chest and rode the crutch by squeezing its pad in my armpit. My stump helped position the crutch for the next step, if needed. It was dicey, but no one ever got hurt. Necessity is the mother of invention, especially for people with a disability.

We moved to shorten my commute and have more room for our growing family. We were in the new house, but not yet fully settled, when it was time to bring Joanna home. We had a room for the little babies to share, while Brendan, who was now eight and whom I had just officially adopted, had his own room in which I built a queen-size, raised platform bed with a desk and play area underneath.

The house was on a one-mile loop road and our driveway was a very steep slope up from our house to the road. Carole had bought a road bike a few years earlier thinking she would like to ride occasionally for fun and exercise, but hadn't really used it much. I was always looking for good ways to build up my leg strength, and I got the idea that maybe biking was something I could do. Now that I was not skiing anything close to one hundred days straight, I really had to worry about my leg being in shape for an annual ski trip to the Rockies or else I would not enjoy it much. Being a perfectionist about skiing, I was quite sensitive to the fact that my technique degraded quite quickly upon the onset of fatigue.

Our driveway was too steep to pedal up, so I crutch-walked to the top of the hill while pushing the bike. I started riding around our circle road and was quite surprised that this worked at all. My pedal pull-up muscles were the ones that became exhausted. We installed rattraps on the pedals so I could pull up and push down. I never wore my prosthesis while riding. It was of no use without a powered knee. In fact, it seemed dangerous. If I fell it could put a ton of leverage on my hip. Since I was just riding around a loop, I left my crutches back at the driveway. Initially, I thought once around the one-mile loop was fantastic, but I quickly worked up to three laps. I got very winded and sweaty from that much of a ride.

About this time I also got back into swimming. I was beginning to get quite out of shape from my years as a graduate student who did nothing but work on a dissertation. All work and no athletics was not like me, but it had been necessary for me to focus entirely on one and only one mission of getting the PhD. It was time to rekindle my athletic side.

I could feel the deleterious effects on my lung, and I vowed never to let myself get out of shape again. I didn't like the feeling of being breathless—it was scary—so I knew I had to become disciplined about exercise again to keep the lung capacity of my remaining lung at or above normal. I had to push myself harder than other people to overdevelop my remaining lung. My missing leg is always obvious to other people, but my missing lung is my invisible disability and it is a constant reminder to me that I had once been given a death sentence. Ultimately, that reminder is what has kept me going back to the gym, the bike, and especially the pool.

I joined a pool close to the Duke campus where, in spite of being full-time at MCNC, I still spent a few half-days each week. I was teaching a seminar or two, had graduate students assigned to me, and was a liaison of sorts between the two institutions.

I got a regular swimming schedule going and met some like-minded guys at the pool with whom I formed a workout group. Noticing that I zigzagged, or fish-tailed, through the water, they came up with the idea of using a flipper. By wearing a swim fin and making the adaptation of kicking in an X-shape, I could compensate for the asymmetry. The fin also helped with flotation of my lower body—the real purpose of kicking in long-distance swimming—so I stayed on the surface better. It felt fantastic to push my lung capacity back up again.

I regained my addiction to the endorphin rush that came with swimming. Our pool was an outdoor pool covered with a bubble during the colder months. The bubble was pretty unacceptable, but we put up with it during the winter. It was such a pleasure to swim again when the bubble came off in the spring. Because I had the experience of swimming competitively as a kid, and because I was willing to work very hard at something, I easily became competitive once again, and I took much pleasure in passing people swimming next to me.

I got a big thrill out of people's reactions to my physical and athletic accomplishments. I enjoyed seeing their reaction when I raced down the pool and executed a clean flip turn, spiked the volleyball over the net, or dropped into a steep ski chute.

It is true that part of what I was doing was showing off. But it's a very different kind of showing off from what I did as a kid. I was making a statement: "Hey, don't think of me as disabled because maybe I can do some things you can't or won't." A person with a disability has a strong desire to move people from their initial reaction of sympathy (which is way too close to pity) to one of respect.

Still, I was reluctant to be seen in public settings—stores, restaurants, movies—without wearing my leg. It invoked staring and an undercurrent of sympathy that was difficult to counteract. All people saw were the crutches. They had no idea what I could really do.

The way I felt when first seen in public without my prosthesis was a stark contrast to how I felt on the ski slope. That was the one place where I did not care if anyone stared. I relished the jaw-drop change in perception that occurred as they saw me first as an amputee with outriggers, and then as a double black diamond skier launching down the steepest chute on the mountain, cruising over the bumps under the lift or floating through an untracked powder field. For me, the psychological benefits of the athletic activities were enormously beneficial. The intellectual prowess of someone who is disadvantaged can be equally beneficial. The bottom line is that we all need ways to excel and stand out from the norm without being judged by our physical appearance or circumstances.

Volleyball was a new discovery. Not picnic volleyball like we played at the wedding. My serious volleyball friends called that "jungle ball." Real volleyball, besides being a fun and social physical activity, became a new way to move people quickly from sympathy to respect. I had played volleyball with two legs, and I had tried it with my leg on once or twice, which was fine for picnic volleyball. But at a PA event at the North Carolina beach one summer day, while I was sitting on the sand watching the game, someone challenged me to do it much more seriously without my leg on.

I did what I always did when presented with a challenge: I met it head on. That day in the sand of a North Carolina beach, I developed a unique volleyball technique using one crutch. On my left side, I used a standard long crutch, which kept my right hand free. With that hand I served, passed, bumped, and even spiked the ball. I hopped around the court leaning on the one crutch, but for a shot that seemed out of reach, I stretched out the crutch horizontally to dig the ball out just before it hit the sand. Players on the opposing team would think the shot was done and relax, but then with my crutch four feet out in front of me, I would pop the ball up just before it hit the ground. In this way, I played four-man volleyball in the sand. I never whacked anyone with my crutch as I dived for an errant shot. I never used the crutch for spiking the ball either; my spikes were always one-handed, but they were strong, and I could jump high enough above the net to make them effective.

One afternoon later that summer, Carole called me at my office, which was south of Durham in Research Triangle Park, to tell me her group from a medical office in Durham was having an impromptu after-work picnic and that there would be volleyball. I said that sounded great, but I did not have my stuff with me, so I asked Carole to bring it to the picnic site. She grabbed my crutches, my one-legged shorts, and my gym shoe. I met her at the picnic and started to change into my stuff when I realized she had brought the wrong shoe. Carole was born with the left-right mix-up gene, but even after all those years together, she also just could not remember which leg I was missing. While relaxing on the sofa watching TV, for example, she would often forget on which side of me to sit so that she could touch the real me and not some wood or metal facsimile of me. I couldn't bear to miss playing a game of volleyball, so I just used my work shoe instead of a sneaker and off we went.

I was working hard at my career. Yes, my "career." Something that implied a future, as did the kids and Carole. I was starting to believe I really was going to be sticking around.

Difficult MCNC politics and Joanna's arrival encouraged me to make a major switch. I went full-time at the university, back in my old department, as a professor of computer science. I had been an adjunct member at the university, but they had been recruiting me for a while to come back full-time. I switched my positions around to be part time at MCNC while teaching and doing research full-time at Duke.

Being a professor was a job that allowed me to be home with the kids a lot. I enjoyed being a dad. We had a nice house, a dog, a cat, a large yard, and three kids running around. I decided I had time for a serious hobby, too, and picked furniture building. Harkening back to a shop class I had taken in junior high, which I had loved, I wanted to learn how to build fine furniture. I had built my first pair of speakers in eighth grade, and I had worked on some wood projects with my mom. I had also built a giant platform bed for Brendan's room and a few bookcases. I purchased a number of "how to" books and started buying serious shop tools. I turned the garage into a shop. North Carolina is furniture Mecca, so I had access to all the furniture hard woods I could want: walnut, ash, maple, and cherry.

After several years and many projects—including a blanket chest, a corner cupboard, and more bookcases—I was finally ready for the biggie. I decided to build an eight-drawer dresser from solid cherry for Carole. Not just cherry, but rough-with-the-bark-still-on-it cherry. I planed and squared the boards; I hand-cut the dovetails; I tongue-and-grooved the back panels; I spent a week per drawer hand-fitting it until it slid in smoothly. The dresser had not one piece of metal in it. Not even nails or screws. The whole project took a year of exacting, painstaking labor. I certainly could never have made a living this way. But it remains one of her prize possessions as her one and only dresser in our bedroom.

Our life revolved around the kids. Carole was home full-time, and I was home a lot, allowing me to spend plenty of time with the children when they were little. I built a commercial-quality wooden swing set, climbing apparatus, sandbox, and tire swing in the back-yard. My workshop looked out at the yard so I could see the kids all the time when they were playing.

After three years, initially as an adjunct faculty and two more as a full-time assistant professor, I discovered several emerging issues in academia. I was a junior faculty member, yet had—by far—the most graduate students. Students liked my projects and they liked the hands-on attention they got from me. It caused resentment from other more senior faculty members who provided less interesting projects and left graduate students to fend mostly for themselves. At the same time, the chairman made a strong proclamation: we were not doing a sufficient job at undergraduate teaching, he said, and from now on the most senior faculty would double down on teaching, while junior faculty would focus more on their research in order to get tenure. As he announced this, I thought, *Great, I can focus on research and do a better job with my large gaggle of graduate students.* Teaching graduate student seminars meant killing two birds with one stone: getting credit for teaching a course, while at the same time advancing my research agenda. However, as my thoughts drifted to the exciting projects I could take on without the more onerous task of teaching undergraduates, the chairman went on to announce, "The only exception to this policy of junior faculty not teaching undergrads is Jothy." *What?* I thought, *Why me? Why was I being singled out this way? Was I being punished?* It was supposed to be a compliment. Because I was deemed so enthusiastic and such a well-liked teacher, I would "get" to teach the very basic introductory computer science course for non-science majors. But to me this was much worse than teaching courses for undergraduate computer science majors.

The course the chairman wanted me to teach was widely referred to as "Computer Science for Poets." I resisted. I complained. It sounded horrible. The chairman's only solace to me was the lecherous comment, "Hey, at least you'll enjoy the attractive co-eds in the class." These non-science majors—male and female—just trying to eke out a science credit, were not at all interested in computers or anything I had to say. It was a struggle just to keep them in their seats. I had to come up with creative ways to keep them from coming just to see if there was a pop quiz and then walking right back out the door when they learned I was just lecturing. One method I used involved a bunch of two-liner off-color jokes that I knew would appeal to twenty-somethings. Neither line in isolation was inappropriate. I began my lecture with the one-line setup to the joke. Then I would lecture about programming, computers, and technology for an hour or so. At the very end, just before I adjourned class, with no fanfare, I blurted out the punch line, seemingly out of context. I found it amazing that this silly trick worked. Every day, if I started to leave without saying the punch line, the students would jump up and beg me to finish the joke—the only reason they had hung on during my "dreadfully boring" lectures. And these were Duke students!

Having to teach "Computer Science for Poets" to a bunch of unmotivated students got me to question whether I was in the right place doing the right thing. I also got to thinking about my time as a student, remembering that the faculty I respected most and learned best from had had real-world practical experience. It seemed I was being a hypocrite on that score. The straw that broke the camel's back for me was wanting to build real parallel computers—my main area of research—with my graduate students; but if we were going to get these systems out for others to use, we needed to be able to maintain them and get the word out (i.e., marketing). That required full-time staff to test, maintain, and document what we built, as well as people to go around "spreading the word" and, of course, selling. Other universities were doing that, but it went too much against the grain at theoretically-oriented Duke.

I was getting an itch. I didn't yet know enough to identify it for what it was—the entrepreneurial itch.

Perhaps there is a gene for entrepreneurship. If so, I had it. Maybe being an entrepreneur is just another hard, risky thing—like skiing—and therefore I was drawn to it. To step out of academia and into a world of building real things, I knew I needed to go to a startup, but there were no such things at that time in North Carolina. There were only two options: Boston or Silicon Valley. California seemed very foreign to someone from Ohio like Carole, who was petrified of earthquakes. So first, I looked hard at Boston. The two other members of my Three Musketeers graduate student group had the same idea and were looking at Thinking Machines Corporation in Boston. I did too.

Thinking Machines was building a massively parallel super-computer similar to my research for NASA, but on a much grander scale. Considered a hot company, they were in an old building right on Kendall Square in the heart of Cambridge, near MIT and Boston. It was a super cool company. They had a playroom for employees with beanbag chairs and lots of kid's toys. That was supposed to help foster creativity because it was thought that, in order to be truly creative, adults needed to get back to their inner child. During the workday, whenever a blast of creativity was needed, employees could wander down to the playroom and hang out until that stroke of creativity suddenly hit them. Or someone throwing a toy truck did. Thinking Machines was too crazy of an environment for me, so I kept looking.

I called the only relative I knew in the computer business, my second cousin, Carol Peters. Carol was from Boston and was a major computer geek and bigwig at Digital Equipment Corporation. DEC was the biggest high-tech company in Massachusetts and huge in the Boston suburbs. Carol had recently moved to California to become a senior manager in DEC's Palo Alto Research Center. She had started as a secretary at DEC, and had risen up to become a manager and a director, eventually becoming general manager of an entire product line.

I knew Carol would have plenty of good ideas, and indeed she did. Carol thought my calling her was providence. Here it was that I had been working on massively parallel computing at Duke, I had interviewed at Thinking Machines, and she was life partner with a founder of the next big thing in Massively Parallel Computing, MasPar. Peter Christy, and some other senior guys from DEC, were starting a direct competitor to Thinking Machines in California. They really wanted my recent experience added to the team. I went out there and talked to them. It was only ten guys. I would be joining on the ground floor of a startup—just what I dreamed of doing. In addition, it was extending and commercializing what I had been working on at Duke. A perfect fit. My interview consisted of everyone in the entire company sitting around a table and talking with me for hours. I described my research at Duke on the NASA machines and how I had purchased and programmed commercial supercomputers to simulate the single-board computers I hoped to build. The job at MasPar was mine if I wanted it.

It was clear now what I needed to do and, reluctantly, Carole agreed. She was so adventuresome and so supportive of me that she was willing to give up the great job she had gone back to when Joanna turned two and our deepening roots in a place we loved, to go to a new, strange place that she was sure would fall into the ocean any day.

SEVEN

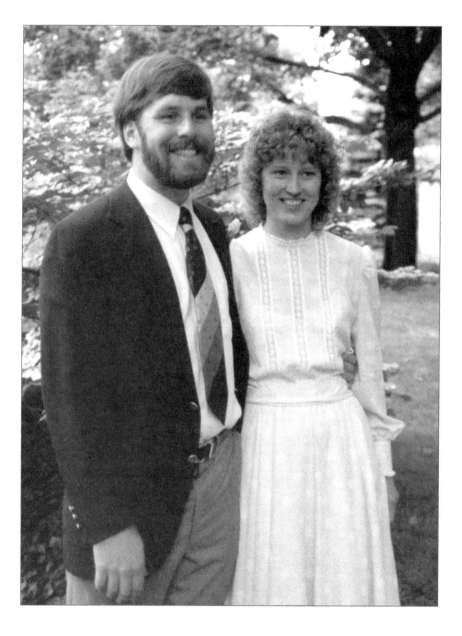

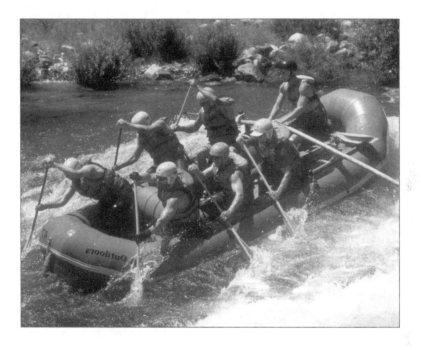

RISKY BUSINESS

As soon as there is life, there is danger.

— Ralph Waldo Emerson, poet

Courage is like love; it must have hope to nourish it.

— Napoleon Bonaparte, French emperor

Perpetual optimism is a force multiplier.

— Colin Powell, general, former U.S. Secretary of State

Moving to California—always an eventful step—was a very big deal after ten years of living comfortably in North Carolina, especially when your wife was an Ohioan who thought only of earthquakes when thinking of California. Carole was otherwise very freethinking and adventuresome and had rebelled a lot against her Ohio and Catholic roots. She was the only one in her family to have left home to attend college, was divorced, thought women should be allowed to be priests, believed in birth control, defended a woman's right to abortion, was vehemently opposed to the death penalty, and thought smoking pot should be decriminalized—to name just a few of the causes Carole championed.

Within two months of my starting at MasPar, we planned to go off for a week of whitewater rafting on the Rio Grande with the river company for which my dad now worked. Four years previously, Dad had quit being a doctor at age fifty-three and had enrolled in law school. He never talked about it, but we all suspected he carried some guilt for not diagnosing my bone cancer earlier. Even if I had been diagnosed in October instead of January, they still would have amputated my leg and the metastasis in my lung would probably still have had time to form. No one—especially me—ever blamed him, but he had his own demons driving him. He was also driven by a great injustice he saw with some shyster lawyers taking on doctors in questionable malpractice cases and winning huge judgments. This outraged him and, while still a practicing surgeon, he had appeared as an expert witness in several medical malpractice cases that were quite egregious in their zealous prosecution of physicians whom he felt had made largely reasonable decisions.

He lasted ten months as a lawyer and then asked why he had entered a field where he saw a lot of compromised ethics and morals. The firm that employed him didn't fully take advantage of his deep knowledge of medicine in defending medical malpractice cases (the reason he had chosen to practice law in the first place). Dad's next move completely surprised all of us. He decided he would finish his "career" as a whitewater rafting river guide.

He had done a few rafting trips for vacations the last few years, but Carole and I had not yet gotten hooked on rafting by going with him. We had done one trip on our own back in North Carolina on the Chattooga river—the river where the movie *Deliverance* was filmed. This Rio Grande trip would be our first with my dad. We eased the trauma of moving to California to join the startup company by going on vacation and inviting my cousin Carol and her partner Peter, who was my new boss, to come along with us.

Carol—without the 'e'—who had introduced me to Peter and to MasPar, was small, with little arm strength for rowing. Peter was a large man, but he did not have great arm strength either. We were a total of fourteen rafters, each with individual one-man inflatable oar boats. Each of the fourteen boats carried one-fourteenth of the total gear we needed for a week on the river. We carried everything in and out with us, even all our human waste. Nothing was to be left behind. Luckily, I did not have the poop containers in my boat.

Joan was the expedition leader—and Dad's boss—and she had a few crewmembers who helped, not that she needed much help. She ran a very tight ship. She was not even afraid to tell guests to shape up. Best of all, she was a gourmet cook at a camp stove. She effortlessly baked a cake in a Dutch oven fashioned out of rocks buried in a hole in the ground.

Rafting was a great sport for me and a critical next rung on the ladder of building self-confidence and exceeding my and other's expectations. Outside of our boats, I was on crutches, so that somewhat limited what I could carry. Being in a boat not only leveled the playing field, but tipped it in my direction. I had rowed plenty in Maine as one of my forms of recovery. I had strong arms and my one leg had plenty of strength for the rowing motion. I could more than keep up with everyone else on the trip. When we were in the boats, everyone forgot I had one leg and one lung. Even me. Yet it was still a big psychological win to do something physical—with no disadvantages at all—as well as, and maybe, just maybe, better than those around me who were considered "normal."

Fourteen boats can easily stretch out over the river for several miles. Joan was always in front, and that was an iron rule. The weakest rowers naturally tended to drift farther and farther to the back. That was where my cousin Carol always was. I, on the other hand, pressed hard at the front. A combination of innate curiosity and competitiveness always had me wondering what was around the next bend—and wanting to be the very first to see it. Joan gently chastised me not to pass her boat, but I kept pushing the envelope anyway. Finally, she came up with an idea for dealing with both the laggards at the back of the line and me in one fell swoop.

Joan decided Carol was too far behind, and she sent me back (upstream) to clip onto Carol's boat and pull her past the other twelve boats to the front. Off I went upstream like an eager puppy chasing a stick. I passed my wife, my parents, Carol's partner (my boss Peter), and all the others to go get Cousin Carol. She was thrilled at the towing idea, as she wanted a rest. Now I was pulling her boat's dead weight, with her in it, and re-passing all the other boats, but this time I was going downstream. I got back to Joan in about half an hour and unclipped Carol's boat so she could start rowing herself again. Inevitably, over the course of the next couple of hours, Carol gradually drifted again to the very back of the line, once again stretching Joan's boat caravan out too far. Joan commanded me to go back upstream to get Carol again and I happily complied. This happened three or four times during the course of each rafting day. Joan hoped this ritual would tire me out and dampen my annoying and relentless pushing on her at the front.

When we camped for the night, Joan had lots of strict rules. One was that no one swam in the river, since the current was strong and she did not want to have to run any daring rescue operations. She made a rare exception for me, however, as she continued to desperately look for ways to tire me out. I was allowed to swim upstream from our camp. Swimming against the current and wearing a life jacket meant I would barely move relative to the shore. Still, it was a lot of additional exercise, and did finally accomplish Joan's goal of tiring me out. The combination of rowing, collecting and towing Carol, swimming, crutch walking all over camp, and carrying my share of loads while on crutches all made it a very arm-focused seven days. Additionally, almost every day we hiked up into the canyons along the river.

On one five-mile hike, I came down the trail pretty fast. If I did a tiny hop after my foot came down, it gave my arms a little more time to get a really long crutch stride going. All I saw were rocks, sticks, and dirt. Just after I'd passed an innocent looking arrangement of rocks, I heard a ruckus behind me. It turned out I had just missed a curled up rattlesnake warming himself in the trail. I had never seen him; his camouflage was so good. A bite on my one leg would have been quite a disaster out in the desert where there was no road access. On future walks, I was much more attentive to the trail ahead of me; in fact, suddenly every rock looked like a rattlesnake to me.

Each day we hit one Class IV rapid as the river went into and came out of fairly steep-walled canyons. The roar could be heard long before it could be seen—the thunder before the lightning. My first impression was that the river just seemed to disappear ahead. That was because it suddenly dropped into the rapids. Class IV rapids are officially defined by the American Whitewater Association as "powerful but predictable rapids requiring precise handling in difficult water. Moderate to high risk to swimmers. Group rescue is often required. Advance scouting is often required." We would indeed scout them. Joan lectured us from some rocks looking down at the rapid we were about to tackle. She told us where to go, where to paddle hard, and what to avoid. Since these were oar boats, we flipped our normal orientation and approached rapids feet first so the rower could see everything coming at them. Each of us was completely on our own. No one else could mess up your line through the rapids, but on the other hand, if you messed up there was only yourself to blame. The oars gave a lot of control and power to slow the boat and to shift from side to side to avoid obstacles in the river.

Joan let me swim, again with a life jacket, through one of the Class IVs after taking my boat through it. That was a huge thrill and a bit scary at the same time. I had to time my breaths carefully as I went from one wave and through a trough to the next wave, all the while being pulled by underwater currents.

That was it; I was now hooked on whitewater rafting. I also had newfound respect for my dad who was having the time of his life on these trips to the Green, Colorado, and Rio Grande Rivers.

Back at MasPar, I quickly got the feel for the culture of a startup company, and I liked it a lot. We were a small, focused, driven, intense team with tight deadlines and long hours. We worked twelve- to fourteen-hour days, six days a week. No one told anyone how to do his or her job. The first crew at a startup has to be self-directed and self-driven. Everyone is just "figuring it out." Like at many startups, no one had done this before, so there was no model to follow. The intensity was infectious. We were creating something from nothing but our own imaginations. The boss brought donuts on Saturday mornings and carefully counted how many were eaten to get an idea of who was committed enough to come in on Saturday.

Our little software team—including Jon Becher, my best graduate student from Duke, who later would become CEO of the company—grew and we started to create working systems. Real working systems built straight from our brains. This was why I had left the university. It was exciting to see our counterpart hardware team developing never-before-created hardware while my software team matched their efforts with a suite of tools to develop code to run on the hardware. We had only simulators (software that behaved as the hardware would when it was fully running) for the first year. I thought the hardware team was really brilliant, and Tom Blank, the overall architect, the most brilliant. Our software team had to modify the UNIX operating system, build compilers and other programming tools, and then also build some applications using the new machines to do really difficult things (like search for a text string in one thousand different New York Times articles simultaneously) that could not be done with standard computers.

Tom, a top swimmer at Stanford when he was in college, introduced me to the Santa Clara swim center where many Olympic athletes train. It was an outdoor fifty-meter pool, which I had never seen before. Tom was much faster than I was, so it was good to swim with him and have him push me. I refused to make excuses; I would try to compete with anyone regardless of how many legs they had.

Our MasPar staff, especially Jon and I, got fanatic about volley-ball. We set up a league and created a great sand court in which to play. I perfected the crutch digs and my spikes over the net, as well as teamwork; it was so much more fun than jungle volleyball. We worked well as a team, and there was a good bump-set-spike sequence on every volley. We played at least once a week. We all enjoyed the reactions of teams from other companies against which we played for the first time. They had no idea what to expect. *Would they hurt this poor one-legged guy? Would this be a silly lopsided game? Isn't it great he's out here trying to participate, but won't it ruin our game?* I didn't mind it because soon enough they changed their attitudes and worried if my next spike was going to be right into one of their foreheads. Jon was the best player on our team, not just because he was the best spiker, but also because he was the best hustler and the most willing to sacrifice his body (at the risk of injury) to get the shot. Like many people, his approach to sports was a reflection of his approach to every other endeavor, which is why he ultimately became the CEO of MasPar.

Selling one of our new supercomputers to a real customer was both scary and fulfilling. Scary because something that came out of our brains was now a big, refrigerator-size thing upon which someone was deciding to spend their hard-earned money. The process of selling something that my team or I invented and built has always awed me. Those products on shelves that people buy, they were made by really brilliant people, not me. I knew too much about the things that I built—including all the warts and flaws. This was true when I built furniture or fancy wooden briefcases in my home wood shop and it was true when my team built software. The thought of someone choosing to buy my product was inconceiv-able. I have never lost my awe of this phenomenon.

Within a year of moving to California, we had the big one Carole—the Midwestern Ohio girl who always feared California would fall off into the Pacific—had dreaded. In fact, it was the biggest earthquake in more than fifty years. Its epicenter, under a mountain called Loma Prieta, was four miles from our house. It was a 7.1 on the Richter scale and happened on October 17, 1989, at 5:04 p.m., one of those dates and times I will never forget. Much of the country remembers it as well because it struck in Oakland at the beginning of game three of the World Series between the Oakland A's and the San Francisco Giants. Of the twelve houses on our street, nine were severely damaged and two were completely destroyed. The destroyed houses were shaken right off their foundations, flattened like cardboard boxes, and thrown down the hill to land in the ravine at the bottom. The houses with the dramatic views up on the highest ridges were the worst off. The ridges were severely shaken, which whipsawed the houses perched on them back and forth in violent motions. So much for their beautiful views.

When the quake occurred, Carole was getting ready to leave work at the Santa Cruz health department. She worked just one town over from where we lived in Scotts Valley, which was up the hill from Silicon Valley. The kids were outside for after-school care at their elementary school. When the quake hit and the trees started rustling, the adults put all the kids under picnic tables. They were probably the safest people in the Santa Cruz Mountains. I was at work down in Sunnyvale in the heart of Silicon Valley, and when the quake came, the whole building felt like it was adrift on an ocean, with long slow swells under us. I jumped up and stood in my office doorway. I started to get vertigo from the very visible slow rolling waves coming through the building. I could see the next wave coming at me through the cement slab floor. The supposedly solid concrete floor strangely looked as liquid as the ocean on a calm day.

Because of the way this earthquake bounced its waves off the deep bedrock, Sunnyvale was spared much damage. The wave passed deep under us; we never even lost power. However, I could not get through on the phone lines, so I had no idea what was happening with my family. TVs worked and we quickly started to see what was happening around the bay. The TV stations were mostly from San Francisco and San Jose, so they focused on those areas and did not immediately notice that the biggest impact was in Santa Cruz near the epicenter.

We were watching the TV as the station sent out their helicopter to take the first pictures. At first, all it showed was a few fires. But then it scanned the Oakland Bay Bridge, and the camera literally did a double-take as it passed the broken section of the bridge. An entire portion of the upper deck had broken free and hinged down to rest one end on the lower deck, while the other end remained attached above. Cars had dropped down to the lower deck when the section of the deck they were driving on had fallen to a forty-five-degree angle. The camera next started to scan the other side of the bay. The double deck of I-880 looked strange. From a distance, it looked lumpy and not tall enough. As the camera got closer, we saw that its entire upper deck roadway had fallen onto the lower deck, crushing all the rush-hour cars on it. That incident alone killed more than sixty people in a frighteningly horrible way. For years afterward, most bay area drivers, including us, never stopped under an overpass when stop-and-go traffic inched along a freeway.

While witnessing all this destruction on TV, I was worried most about my side of the hills. I was still unable to get through on the phone, and Highway 17 over the hill was shut down tight. I stayed with Jon at his apartment, and later that night the phones started to work. I was able to find out that Carole had managed to get to the kids and then, by driving on back roads and winding around downed redwood trees, had gotten back up to our house. What they found was an intact house with a huge mess inside and some safe but scared Golden Retrievers out in their pen. All the kitchen shelves had disgorged their newly canned tomatoes, beans, berries, and more. In the center of the kitchen was a pile two feet high of broken glass, can tops, and tomato goop. There was no power for days, so this had to be cleaned up by flashlight. Luckily, when you live in those hills, you have a generator, you heat with wood, and you have gravity-fed water tanks with huge capacity. We were self-sufficient for a week or more.

Meanwhile, I was still over the hill in Silicon Valley squirming that I could not get home. Highway 17 was in horrible shape. The center cement Jersey barrier was smashed in more than a thousand places. Giant redwood trees were downed on both sides of the highway, and huge chunks of tire-slicing asphalt roadway had heaved up, creating impassible sections.

I was unperturbed. In the morning, I drove right up to the entrance of the highway in my VW Jetta. The state trooper blocking the entrance must have seen a maniacal look in my eyes. He allowed me to pass, but made it clear that I was "on my own."

A Jetta is not a four-wheel drive all-terrain vehicle by any stretch of the imagination. I went up the road on the normal side and found it impassible. I went back down and tried the lanes on the other side of the barrier going in the other direction. Going the wrong way didn't matter because I might as well have been on the face of the moon. No one else was trying what I was trying. Some sections of the road had landslides. One place I passed was clear, but only an hour later it got buried under forty feet of mud. In some places I tried to pass roadway that was raised a foot above the adjacent roadbed. In other places, I had to go way up the side of a hill to get around a redwood tree. I finally made it after a tortuous two-hour drive. Everyone was home and it was great to be there all together.

We tolerated aftershocks that came fast and furious in the 4 to 4.5 range. Not small, but not damaging. I got into cleanup mode. We were in that mode for four days before we got the place into some semblance of order. A generator powered the critical parts of the house. We cooked on the wood stove. Everyone was so freaked out by the aftershocks—including our two Golden Retrievers—that we all just camped out on the floor near the wood stove for several nights.

Our neighbors were not nearly as lucky as we were. Brendan was dog sitting for the neighbors while they were down salvaging their boat in the Caribbean, which had been damaged by Hurricane Hugo the week before. Theirs was the house that had completely gone down the side of the hill into the ravine. The dog was stressed, but okay. Luckily, his doghouse survived and we could calm him down in that.

Another neighbor's house straight up the hill from ours was okay, but their deck collapsed and their pool went over the side of the hill in one piece. I spent many weekends helping Mike Smith rebuild his two thousand-square-foot deck. I learned from this experience, and I quickly put lips on all our shelves, bolted all of the bookcases to the walls, and tied down large, fragile things like TVs.

Travel to Sunnyvale was a nightmare for more than a month. Highway 17 was closed to everyone who didn't live right on it, as we did. The State Police created caravans of one hundred cars, with one cop at the front and one in back. The whole caravan snaked back and forth from the correct side of the highway to the wrong side and back, depending on where the road was passable. A one-way trip took nearly two hours. They worked on repairs twenty-four hours a day, but it wasn't until Thanksgiving that Highway 17 was open in both directions.

The Santa Cruz Mountains are a great area for outdoor activities, especially during the summer. We hiked a lot, joined by our good friend, Jon. Jon was not just my former graduate student and a MasPar colleague; he was part of our family in California, just as he had been back in North Carolina. On one of our many hikes, we saw a sign for "Skyline to the Sea." It's a trail that goes from the two thousand-foot ridgeline of the Santa Cruz range all the way to the ocean, a distance of about twelve miles. Like most of the trails through those hills, it was a twisty, but mostly gentle, downward slope toward the ocean. We decided to spend an afternoon walking that trail to the ocean, where a bus would take us back into Santa Cruz to our parked car. I wore my usual moleskin on my sides and sports tape on my hands to survive a crutch hike that long.

My speed hiking with crutches is comparable to other walkers. However, we had kids with us who couldn't make it all the way. (At that time, Brendan was in junior high school and Zac and Joanna were in preschool.) Jon, Carole, and I took turns carrying one of the little ones on our shoulders. Carrying an extra thirty to forty pounds on my shoulders, after being tired already, made for a most memorable hike. First, my arms started to feel normal fatigue. Then a period of muscle pain occurred, which gradually transitioned to numbness. If I stopped, they stiffened up. I knew when I stopped for good they would ache for several days. Just as we got to where we could see the road and the ocean, we also saw the last bus of the day just pulling away from the stop where we were supposed to catch it. Luckily, one hiker from our group was farther ahead and got the attention of the driver, who waited for him to get on but would not wait for the rest of us. That was okay since our advance scout came back for us in the car.

Another hike we often did was much farther south at a place called Pinnacles. It was an ancient volcano site that was smack dab on the middle of the San Andreas fault and had been split in half and separated by the slippage in that fault. We climbed on the western half of the volcano. The eastern half is 195 miles farther south. In the 23 million years since the Neenach Volcano had erupted, the fault has slid the western part of California 195 miles north. It made for very interesting hikes. This one was filled with steel ladders and tricky ropes to get over some very steep terrain. To climb a ladder, I looped my crutches into my belt and used my arms and one leg (occasionally using my stump to stabilize). The really tricky part was helping our seventy-five-pound Golden Retriever, Lazarus, which I sometimes did by putting him on my shoulders, legs hanging down on either side of my neck, while I climbed the ladder. He was calm and trusting enough to put up with that, and my arms were able to pull my weight plus his up a ladder. Fortunately the kids needed less and less help as they had become very good hikers.

We had lived in California for more than five years before we made it to Yosemite Valley. Vernal Falls is formed by the Merced River flowing over a large rocky plateau and tumbling more than a thousand feet to the valley floor. It then turns into a Class IV runnable river out of Yosemite on its way out of the Sierras and through the Central Valley (first as the American River and then as the Sacramento River), emptying into San Francisco Bay.

The hike from the valley floor up to the top of the falls is one of the more popular hikes in Yosemite. The lower part of the trail is always crowded. Even novice hikers can make the lower trail, but then the Mist Trail turns into a giant 317-foot staircase of wet, slippery rocks up the side of the giant falls. The crowds thin out at this point, but there are still many people who think they can make this climb. I always got into a Zen-like state to do it. As usual, I thought of it as another athletic event and wanted to set some sort of record. I blasted up these steps two at a time with my left leg and quickly pulled the crutches up behind me to get ready for the next two-step leg lift. A nice steady rhythm. People who saw me coming would jump to the side to get out of the way of the madman on crutches. Those who didn't see me right away kept climbing with me on their tail until eventually they too jumped out of my way. As I raced to the summit, I was like a north polarized magnet to the hundreds of south polarized climbers, jumping left and right like repelled magnets to let me pass.

This attitude I had developed—this super-aggressive drive to perform at a level higher than others—was a psychological adaptation on my part to overcompensate and prevent that dreaded pity reaction. It's a natural defense mechanism, one born of a disabled person's desire to combat their disability's constant attacks on their self-confidence, self-image, and ultimately, self-esteem. The process I was going through was a healthy voyage of self-discovery that anyone recovering from major trauma or newfound disability needs to go through. I was having my own "Post-Disability Syndrome" just like what Lauro Halstead found when interviewing polio survivors for his *Scientific American* article, "Post-Polio Syndrome," where one said, "Don't let anyone tell you that we just want to be 'normal' like everyone else. We have to be better than everyone else just to break even . . . and that may not be enough."

Carole and I both got very involved with the elementary school as our young ones entered kindergarten and beyond. California was one of the first states where the tax busters wreaked their havoc. Proposition 13, titled the "People's Initiative to Limit Property Taxation," cut off funds from property taxes, and soon the schools were gasping for air. To us, as parents, it was an outrage. The elementary schools were constantly looking for ways to raise extra money. In one swipe, these selfish tax zealots had taken California's public schools from first to forty-ninth in the nation.

Haunted houses at Halloween were a common fundraiser for the schools. I heard about such a fundraiser and wanted to get involved. The first year, I was a worker bee who did random tasks like painting and fastening curtains and props. The organizer was Maureen, a woman with boundless energy and a creative knack for making these haunted house experiences amazing and scary. Every year she set records for how much money the event raised for the schools.

The second year, I was a scary zombie. I stood very still, facing the wall, until kids neared my area; then I jumped out, screaming at them and scaring them to death. After Maureen learned about my leg, she began to fashion some very warped ideas for how to use me in the third year's haunted house.

That's when things got really debauched and twisted. Maureen decided the theme was going to be a torture chamber centered on me as the star attraction. Visitors made their way through the haunted house, where each room focused on a different method of torture—each with increased levels of intensity.

They reserved me for the last and, by far, scariest room. This room contained a headless Steve Dunlop (the father of my daughter's best friend), where it looked like his detached head was sitting on a bale of straw. It was a nice trick. If you didn't look too closely, it was pretty darn convincing. Steve was funny with his head attached to his body, and he was absolutely hilarious with his head sitting on a bunch of straw.

Also in this room was the man on the rack. He was my kids' favorite teacher, John Magliato. Strung up on the wall moaning and straining against his shackles, he added nicely to the aura of torture in this room. Then came the centerpiece—me. I was lying on a table with a nasty torturer woman standing over me with a huge axe that was to come down and cut off my leg. I was supposed to be a prisoner who was not telling the torturer what she wanted to know, and supposedly chopping off my leg would get me to confess.

The trick was especially convincing because they took one of my old discarded artificial legs, made it look all bloody, and attached stuff to the socket that looked like pieces of fresh muscle tissue. The entire leg was dressed just like my other leg, with a rip in the pants at the top of the socket. The torture lady's axe was attached to a very thin wire that went through pulleys behind her and was ultimately attached to the foot of my prosthesis. When she brought the axe down to chop off my leg, the wire pulled the leg away from the rest of me and she hit the table hard with the axe blade, without a real part of me in the way. As the axe struck, I would squirm and make my stump spasm as if it had just been cut. Little, fake, bloody, muscle pieces pinned to my stump would flap around, as did those attached to the prosthesis. I admit it was very gross.

As people walked from room to room in our haunted house, what they saw got progressively worse, and it was all so realistic that they came into this last room having reached a plateau of abject terror. Headless Steve would greet them, Chained John would writhe in pain, and then the axe lady would cut my leg off. When they saw our stunt, clearly not faked, many of them lost it.

Some ran at full speed out of the building. Some were the scientific types who had to figure out the trick; they came close to the table looking for where my leg must be bent and tucked under the table, but they could find evidence of no such trickery. That made them feel quite faint, and some of them then also ran screaming from the building. It was so convincing we actually got into trouble. The complaint for weeks afterward was that a school fundraiser should be more consistent with the "values" of the schools themselves, and since the schools would never directly condone torture, or should I say, "pretend torture," perhaps we should not be doing the event in association with the schools. Of course, they had no problem accepting the enormous donation to the schools that our torture-filled haunted house had earned.

MasPar had built and sold one hundred machines during my four years with them. That is impressive by supercomputer standards. Still, I was starting to feel some dissatisfaction. Customers finding issues—bugs—in our software angered and embarrassed me. If it was a serious bug, we provided each customer with a patch to install over the existing software. With only one hundred machines in the field, that was not terribly difficult. I knew if we had sold thousands, that would not work (no Internet distribution existed at this point), and so I wanted to figure out why we didn't have more robust, less buggy software. That eventually led me to my next job.

I was fully vested in my stock options and feeling an itch to find out how to build really high-quality software that wouldn't constantly need patches to fix bugs. I started asking everyone I could find who they thought was building the highest-quality software on the planet. They all answered with the same name: Borland. It just so happened Borland was a short two miles from my house, on the same side of the mountains. If I went to work for Borland, not only could I learn from the best, but I could also avoid one of the nastiest commutes in the entire San Francisco Bay area.

Borland was a big company, and its products depended fundamentally on Windows PCs. If I was nervous about going to a big company, I was despondent about going to a company that used PCs running horrid Microsoft software as opposed to workstations running my beloved UNIX. I'd enjoyed an intimate, unbroken relationship with UNIX since I entered graduate school twelve years before, but I was going to have to overcome my prejudice if I wanted to learn, from the inside, how to build the best, most bug-free, software. And I was determined to do just that.

When I first joined Borland, I was hired to manage a small team responsible for Borland's debugger. Like any debugger, Borland's customers used it to track down errors in their programs. It was the most widely used and sophisticated debugger available.

My new team was at each other's throats and completely dysfunctional. What the team needed most was help getting back on schedule. To do that, they needed to first fix all the known bugs. (Yes, even debuggers have bugs in them.) Even though I was the manager, I dove in to find and fix bugs in the code. I helped get things on track and made the team feel very successful. We shipped our product shortly thereafter, declaring a major success.

In the process of leading and working side-by-side with the team, I was shocked to find that there were no books describing how debuggers work. More than two million people used our debugger daily. Wouldn't many of them like to know how the thing worked? If the only way for me to learn how to build a debugger was to look at the source code and ask around, shouldn't someone write a book to make it easier for the next poor guy trying to do what I was doing?

With my initial notes from building the MasPar debugger and my new experience with Borland's debugger, I set off on a six-year project to write the first book on debuggers. The marketing department at Borland helped me find a publisher who was interested. When I was thinking of a name for the book, my kids and I came up with "Debuggers Demystified." We loved it. It had a nice ring.

When I proposed it to the publisher they said, "Oh no, we can't use '*Anything* Demystified.' That's taken."

"What do you mean it's taken?" I asked.

"Well, publishers can own a formula for a title, like '*XYZ* for Dummies' is taken, and no one else can use that."

"Okay," I said, "Give me an example of the Demystified formula in use."

"*Mushrooms Demystified*," they said matter-of-factly.

"But do you really think anyone will confuse mushrooms with debuggers?" I asked.

"Doesn't matter, the whole template is taken. You have to think of something different."

"Do you have a suggestion?" I asked.

"Well sure. Let's just say what it's about. Let's call it 'How Debuggers Work?'" And so that was it. Dreadful but descriptive. In 1996, I did it. I published *How Debuggers Work* with a major publisher and it could be purchased on Amazon.com. It went on to sell more than five thousand copies and was translated into Japanese.

Borland was a milestone in my career. It was the most focused and intense environment I had ever worked in, even more so than MasPar. People were committed. They were very customer-focused. Everyone knew Microsoft was after us, so there was a strong dose of healthy paranoia that we could be snuffed out in an instant. We had to be smart and good, as well as fast, just to stay alive. It made the environment intense, and I loved it.

Borland's success and its genius was its people. There was a brief time when it attracted the best and the brightest. People worked there because it was the most innovative company, and it built the best-quality products in all of Silicon Valley, if not the world. The unappealing "get rich quick" philosophy came to the valley much later. When the smartest people are motivated for the right reasons, when they are very clear about who their customers are and what they want, great products result and the company remains great, for at least a little while. There were other divisions of Borland that were not healthy. I lived through tumultuous times during which it went through five CEOs, had seven layoffs—one involving more than thirty percent of the workforce—and lost most of the value of the stock. Until the end, however, Borland kept the best people, maintained the highest quality and innovativeness of its products, and held on to its customers. To this day, I have never seen a more loyal customer base, and whenever I see a former Borland employee, I know they are among the best.

I got promoted and was again a VP. I had first been a VP at age twenty-six back in North Carolina and thought I was the bee's knees, which I manifested by wearing those pretentious suspenders. I now knew that a jump into the executive ranks with no real practical experience had done me no favors. Ten years later, now at thirty-six, being a VP really meant something. I had actually earned it this time.

One of the great things about kids is that they always know how to humble their parents. The day of my promotion, I was feeling pretty full of myself. I called home to tell Carole the news and that I was bringing home a bottle of champagne. As I walked in the door, my innocent little daughter, who was only ten, hit me with, "Welcome home your royal VP-ness," at which point Carole and I laughed so hard we had trouble staying in our chairs.

The whitewater rafting trip down the Rio Grande had given me the bug to do more of it. I liked the thrill. I had a strong taste for challenges and danger. I liked the speed of the water, the physical challenge of paddling and staying in the raft, and the requirement for technical skill to do it well. In addition, I loved the fact that I was able to excel at something that was very challenging for people with two legs. California is heaven for whitewater rafting. The three forks of the American River, the Tuolumne, Merced, Stanislaus, and California Salmon are all runnable rivers each spring and early summer. Some are Class III, some IV, and just a few had Class V rapids. Class VIs are considered unrunnable and can kill you. Class Vs are no picnic either. The official American Whitewater Association classification description for Class V is "extremely long and/ or violent rapids, often containing large, unavoidable obstacles, holes, steep banks, and turbulent water. Rescues are often difficult for experts. Advance scouting may be difficult."

Here, our boats were mostly six-man or eight-man rafts with a guide who sat in the back. The front two positions, called "points," are really important. I always sat at right point. That's because I had experience, and due to having only the left leg to hold me in the raft, I had to sit on the right side. When sitting on the outer tube of the boat, a two-legged paddler twists a little at the waist and braces their legs inside the boat, against the tube and the thwarts that run side-to-side across the boat. Since I have only the left leg to get inside the boat, I don't have to twist at the waist. When my single leg is well braced, I am actually as close to secure on my perch as any two-legger. By sitting squarely on the tube facing directly forward, I have a huge power advantage and can apply full strength to my paddle in the water. That, plus the fact that crutch walking and swimming for many years has naturally built up my arm strength, means I have an extra power advantage.

A number of things just fit better for an amputee without a pesky right leg in the way. It means better sitting on a couch with my wife. Where my leg is absent, hers lies comfortably. No crisscrossing legs. It means we can go kayaking with the dog. He lies where my right leg is not. The advantages go on and on. As a one-legged skier, I have no fear of crossing my ski tips. I can get on and off a bike faster since there is nothing to lift over the bike to the other side.

We did a few whitewater-rafting trips as a family. They were fun outings, getting us up into the Sierras and outdoors together. We did the Class III branches of the American River that come down out of the Sierras toward Sacramento, where they merge into a single large river that flows through Sacramento and into San Francisco Bay.

As I got more and more hooked on whitewater, I began to look for a way to push the envelope. The family could not go beyond a Class III, so I decided to form a group that could. I started to recruit other interested people from my colleagues at Borland. We did a trip or two, driving up super early in the day, rafting all day, and then driving home again. A team began to coalesce. Each member naturally found a fixed position in the boat and learned that position and the signals of the others on the team. We began to learn each other's rhythms and strengths. We learned to anticipate what the boat needed to do next even before the guide told us. We found guides who tested our technical skills and taught us more challenging maneuvers. We practiced drills on the river. Some rapids required going straight down, bumping gently on a rock to turn the boat, ferrying straight across the river, going down backwards, and quickly spinning away from a hole. To balance me at right point, we put a big strong guy at left point. He was a former Marine and very big and strong. He needed to be because that twist at the waist cut back his power and he had to balance against me. We became a precision drill team of six guys.

We were ready for the big stuff.

We did the Merced at super high water. It had standing fifteen-foot waves that needed to be hit perfectly straight on or they would roll our boat right over. We did the Tuolumne, which is a very technical Class IV-V river requiring the fanciest maneuvers. One spring, we decided to try the Stanislaus.

It was May. The air was warm, around eighty degrees. We drove up the night before and stayed in the cabin of our Borland colleague, Eli Boling, on Bear Mountain. I drove up in my BMW convertible, top down, with my leg on, wearing moccasins. When we arrived at the road into his subdivision, it did not look right. Where the road was supposed to be was an eight-foot wall of snow. It turns out the entire subdivision never plows all winter and May is still too early for it to have melted. People who live up there use snowmobiles all winter to get to and from their mountainside houses. Eli forgot to tell us this.

We had to park and walk with our stuff. It was a couple of miles up to the house. Moccasins are very slippery on wet spring snow, and my leg just wouldn't behave in these conditions. It was amusing and frustrating at the same time. It would have been worse on crutches, which would have sunk up to my elbows anyway. I slipped and slided, and occasionally wiped out, on the slow route up to the house. The soft snow cushioned my falls, and my compatriots stayed with me so I wouldn't get lost. It was pitch dark by the time we finally made it to the house.

The next morning, several of the team wanted to find an easier and faster way down for me. We found a large wardrobe box, broke it down, and fashioned it into a cardboard toboggan. I sat down on this device; they gave me a push; and off I went. It was a smooth but curvy path down, like a bobsled run, and the makeshift toboggan followed that path perfectly. I had a few minor tumbles along the way, but I made it to the bottom before the others and in a fraction of the time it had taken me on the way up the night before.

The river was nearby and we were there in plenty of time for the put-in. It was a spectacular May day in the Sierras with a crystal clear blue sky and a hot sun. The air was in the eighties, but there were still ice chunks along the banks of the river. As the water had just been released from melting snowpack a few minutes previously, its temperature was only thirty-four degrees. Face shots—where an ice cold wave breaks over your head—would take your breath away, and then you were instantly warm again.

The river was flowing high and fast. It was mostly a Class IV river, with a couple of very technical class Vs. Midway down the river was a Class IV of awesome power. It caught us off guard, and was the first time our team had ever gotten dunked. One guy from another boat was in the water so long that he turned mostly blue as he was buffeted against boats and rocks before we could hoist him back in the boat.

This run prepared us for the most challenging river in California, and one of the toughest in North America—the California Salmon. Most people, even those who know California well, have never even heard of this river. It is in the Trinity Alps Primitive Area, one of the most isolated regions in the state. It is closer to the coast than the Sierras, due west of Mt. Shasta, way north of San Francisco, and not far from the Oregon border. It drains the Sawtooth Glacier, the only glacier in California's coastal range. It's dam-free its entire length, so it depends solely on snowmelt for its flows. The California Salmon has about five Class V rapids and a dozen Class IVs. The first day builds up to a crescendo for an even more intense second day. The ultimate Cal Salmon rapid is "Freight Train," where the river drops seventy-five feet in less than a mile. The entire river turns frothy white side-to-side that entire stretch. Right before Freight Train is a very technical Class IV, aptly named "Last Chance." The two were going to be a real test of our skills. Ominously, my Marine counterpart was not on this trip. He had family commitments and could not join us. So Eli took left point, and while he is a great rafter, he is much smaller than the usual left point guy and was not used to balancing against me.

As we got close to Freight Train, the guides started speaking with higher-pitched voices; it was clear they were scared. It was vital that no one swam through Freight Train; the froth makes it almost impossible to get air into your lungs and you would probably die. To prevent swimmers from drifting into it as the result of an incident on Last Chance, the river crew set up ropes across the river and strategically placed kayakers below Last Chance and just before Freight Train.

Last Chance requires taking the boat straight toward a huge rock, which if touched would bounce it into a hole bigger than an SUV. Ideally, the best route is to turn hard right above the rock, skim across the top of the gigantic hole, turn hard left past the hole, and continue straight down between the hole and the riverbank.

The boat in front of ours bumped the first rock, which spun them around and sent them, tail first, straight into the SUV-eating hole. Each rafter popped up quickly and started drifting straight for Freight Train. The kayakers and ropes caught them all in time. The second boat made it past the first rock and tried to skim across the river above the hole, but they, too, were swept into the hole and dumped. Again, all swimmers were safely retrieved before the frightening Freight Train froth.

Our turn. We headed for the huge rock straight downstream. Just above it, the guide started yelling "right turn" and we crisply turned the boat to face across the river without touching the dreaded rock. Now the hole was downriver, just to our left, as we tried to skim above it to the other bank of the river. The guide started screaming "dig, dig, dig," over and over, louder and louder. My adrenalin shot up and I dug in harder than I ever had before. Unfortunately, even though poor Eli did too, I overpowered him. As the guide saw the boat slowly head toward the killer hole, his instinct was of course to yell "dig" louder and many more times, so I responded with even more strength. Everything worked backwards. The harder he told us to dig, the more my overpowering of Eli forced the boat to the left, closer and closer to the dreaded hole. We might have skimmed across perfectly if not for my forcing us directly into the hole. We were all dumped in, pushed down, and with our life vests on making us act like corks, popped back out below that hole in the blink of an eye. The water was cold, so it immediately shocked our systems. The water was also moving fast, so we got pushed down river so rapidly we couldn't get our bearings. Fortunately, we all were snagged by the kayakers and safety lines and taken to shore safely. However, the boat was caught in the hole, which acted like a giant suction on the bottom of the boat. Left alone the boat could have stayed there for hours, with my crutches securely attached to it. It took us half an hour to free our boat and get ready for Freight Train.

In an anti-climactic way, Freight Train turned out to be relatively easy after that. It was such a horrendous rapid that the only way to run it was to aim the boat straight into it and then all drop down to the floor of the boat where we would lock arms to ride straight down the throat of the massive torrent. It funneled us into a narrow slot of unimaginable power and speed only to drop us into a large, quiet pool of still water. Once through, we all just sat there in the bottom of our boat, arms still locked, looking up at the sky, quietly contemplating our mortality.

Years later, when we had moved to the East Coast, I got my son Zac hooked on whitewater too. We did the Dead and the Kennebec in Maine and the Gauley in West Virginia. Zac took the job of left point and we learned to balance against each other. He was strong and fearless about large waves and would lean forward and grimace and bark at fifteen-foot walls of water, as if to dare the river to knock him out of the boat.

With access to the Sacramento River Delta, where waterskiing is a huge activity, I rejuvenated my waterskiing focus. When I was a kid at Lake Temagami, and still two-legged, all we had was a very low-power boat. My dad had no boat driving experience. Getting up took a long time, even with two skis, because the engine was so underpowered. I always liked the thrill of the speed and the feel of being on top of the water. On two skis, I had little to do but track behind the boat and occasionally cross the wake unexcitedly. On one ski, I had a lot more maneuverability to cut back and forth. Two-legged skiers use their back foot for leverage to start the hard cuts. With just the front foot, I steer the ski more than cut it. Eventually I bought my own ski and moved the one boot back so I had more leverage. I just had to learn to twist harder than two-leggers to get the cuts going.

I started to notice a few people barefoot waterskiing in the heavily-traveled Sacramento River Delta waterskiing areas where we always went. Someone noticed my fascination with this rare but impressive feat and said, "A one-legged person could never barefoot water ski." This proclamation—almost a dare—became my next obsession. Years later, I finally found someone who knew how to barefoot and had the right equipment to teach me how to do it. Most importantly, they wanted to see an amputee pull this off.

To learn how to barefoot, you need a fast boat with a side pole. The pole sticks out the middle side of the boat so the people in the boat can talk to you and coach you through the process. This pole has a short ski rope handle attached to it. As a beginner, I wore a padded bodysuit, a cup, a neck brace, and strong nose plugs. The padded suit and cup protected my family jewels and prevented the dreaded water-skiing enema effect. The neck brace offered protection against forward falls of forty-seven miles per hour. The boat dragged me along as I hung from the pole until it got up to speed—a speed that is higher than normal waterskiing by about ten miles per hour. I had to learn how to plane on my back in the padded suit and to hyperflex my foot backward. If any toe bent forward and caught water, it pulled me forward fast and I rolled hard on to my face. By hanging onto the training pole, I could try this dozens of times without falling off and forcing the boat to stop and come around to pick me up. Eventually, I got the feel of planing on my back with my leg up in the air, slowly lowering my leg until my heel dipped into the water, and then carefully rocking forward until I was only on my foot, planing across the water.

At this point, I was barefoot skiing from a pole, but that didn't really count. I wanted to deep-water start, so next I set out to learn how to plane on my back from the end of a long rope behind the boat. I looped my leg up over the rope, making sure my nose plug was secure, and slowly arched my neck and back, letting the water across which I was speeding hit the back of my head. Basically, I used the back of my head to plane across the water. Soon I was able to plane along, bouncing on my back, thanking the inventors of my padded suit. Oh, and thanking the God of the Lakes that no debris was in the way to hit me on the head.

As the boat speed climbed, I shifted to planing on my back with my head and foot up in the air. Just like on the pole, I slowly lowered my heel into the water and rocked forward. After a few tries I eventually got the hang of it. I was up on one foot going forty-seven miles per hour screaming around the river delta for the entire world to see. I was happy and scared at the same time. I knew what Carole knew: this was really dangerous. A small stick in the water at that speed, with no foot protection, could take off a toe. If I lost my big toe, I would not be able to walk at all on crutches or with a prosthesis. I was being incredibly stupid. I shouldn't try anything that threatens my one leg. For days afterward, I had trouble walking due to major bruising to the ball of my foot from the high-speed water pressure. I was hugely satisfied, but unlike most things I took up as new sports, I knew this was a one-time thing. I had done what I set out to do, but I would never try this stupid stunt again.

The only form of heat in our house up in the Santa Cruz Mountains was wood. As we lived in sparsely populated, densely wooded hills, I was determined to get my own wood. There were four problems with that mission. First, the trees were all downhill from the roads where vehicles could be parked and loaded with cut wood. Second, the hills were quite inhospitable to human inhabitants, being densely vegetated with poison oak and infested with rattlesnakes. Third, the footing around the trees was extremely shaky and a severe challenge for an artificial leg. And fourth, it was hot, sweaty work. My leg socket back then was held on strictly with suction. Sweat reduced the friction between the skin and the plastic, resulting in a loss of suction. A safety belt kept it from completely dropping off, but basically my leg was barely secure during these cutting sessions.

No big deal. I adapted. My neighbor, Mike Smith, was equally maniacal about cutting wood for his woodstoves. We built a sled on which to load logs down in a ravine and used a pulley system powered by his truck to pull the loaded sled back up the slope so we could load it into the truck. Now all we had to do was get down into the ravine and cut and split all the wood we wanted.

On one occasion, Mike and I set out to cut a big, downed tree in a deep ravine. I balanced on one end, with Mike at the other. We were careful and experienced chainsaw guys and followed standard safety protocols, but there were close calls just the same. Normally I kept both hands on the saw at all times, but on one cut I had to reach far up over my head and hold myself up with one hand while cutting with the other. The saw went through the branch faster than I expected, and then swung down, with its chain still spinning fast. The heavy saw was moving fast, and with only one available hand, I didn't have enough leverage to stop it. The chain hit my right leg, ripped through my jeans, and cut deeply into the fiberglass of my thigh. Then it stopped. My pants were ruined, my heart was beating through my chest, and Mike was freaking out, but there was no real harm to the saw or my leg—and my good leg was untouched. I had long since learned to keep my artificial leg in front of me when doing this sort of thing. With a few notable exceptions (like barefoot waterskiing), I have always consciously and subconsciously taken great pains to protect my one good leg.

An amputee spends a lot of time with their prosthetist—much more time than most people spend with any doctor or dentist. Prosthetic legs are hard to fit and difficult to keep comfortable. Skin is simply not designed to rub against plastic, with the pressure of one's full body weight, for eighteen hours a day. Plus, artificial legs are not intended to put up with what I demand of mine: miles of walking, kneeling in garden dirt, getting whacked by chainsaws down in ravines, and being pummeled by high-powered air pressure staples. Technology moves pretty fast, however, and there are frequent advancements in prosthetic science that require "guinea pigs" to test them.

Stanford University Rehabilitation Hospital was a leader in prosthetics. With them, I switched early to a new technology for suspension (how the leg is held onto the residual limb or stump). The new technology was designed to solve two big problems with suction suspension. First, suction fails quite easily when there is too much perspiration, or when the leg is struck hard or the toe catches on a step when climbing stairs. Second, skin rubbing against the hard plastic of the socket is a war that the skin always loses. Skin breakdowns are common, as are bleeding and pain. It's a constant fight for comfort. Amputees look like they are walking in pain because they are. That, or their leg is barely hanging on and they need to go to a private place to reattach it.

With the conventional simple suction suspension, I pulled a sock over the stump and used the end of that sock, through a valve hole in the bottom of the leg socket, to pull the stump into the socket. I then pulled the sock all the way out and screwed a valve in the hole to create a vacuum to hold the stump in place.

The new technology designed at Stanford did not use suction, but instead used a strong silicon liner with a pin welded to its tip. To attach the leg, I inverted the liner and rolled it onto the skin of the stump. I then pulled the pin through a hole in the end of the hard socket casing. It fit reasonably tightly, and the close-fitting silicon did not slide against my skin when put under pressure. The stump held in the socket more securely than with suction suspension, while protecting my skin from rubbing.

Getting a new leg was not like getting a crown at the dentist, comprised of one or two visits. It required visits once or twice a month for an entire year. To have a new leg, I needed to see my prosthetist more times than most women visit their OB/GYN to have a new baby. Still it was worth it to me. My new leg was so much more securely suspended, and it never needed adjustment once we got it right. The new knee was better, too—stable and smooth, so I no longer stumbled.

I still walked with a definite limp. No matter what, I will not get rid of that until they build a powered ankle. It is partly due to the way a prosthesis works. I swing the leg forward from behind and, during the swing, the knee straightens out so that when I land the heel on the ground in front of me, the knee is perfectly straight. The mechanics of the knee work by locking when the knee is straight and there is a little load on it from pressure against the foot. The swing forward comes from the hip, since the ankle has no power source. (Advancements are being made in this area, but they are yet to be perfected.) Normal two-legged walking gets most of its energy for the next swing from the ankle push off. Most of the job of a real knee is to act like a break to stabilize the leg as weight is placed on it. A flesh and blood knee is not locked perfectly straight when weight lands on it. The landing on a perfectly straight and locked mechanical knee also contributes to a pronounced limp. Finally, because of the flexion contracture that flexes my stump a little bit forward instead of pointing straight down, the hip does more work and makes for a lessened range of motion.

I had been using a sixty-foot outdoor pool (smaller than a normal twenty-five-yard pool) at a club we joined when we first moved to Scotts Valley. I was swimming fairly regularly, but not pushing it very hard. It kept me in reasonable shape, but there were no events or goals that helped drive me. I introduced Steve Bird, who was part of my debugger team at Borland, to swimming. He struggled to swim even a few lengths, but something in him was driven to get good at this and to get in shape. Within no time, he was swimming as far as I was. He left the company and soon was getting involved in triathlons. Steve and a friend asked me to consider joining a team triathlon event where each of the three people does a different event. I would do the swim. In the ocean. That's dark, cold water with no lane lines to keep the swimmer straight. Even with all the time we spent on lakes, I hadn't done any real swimming in open water. Steve and his friend would do either the cycling or the running leg of the event. I had to get a little experience with open water swimming before I could do this, so I joined a weekend morning group that swam in the ocean near Santa Cruz.

It was totally intimidating. The water was dark, and my imagination went a bit wild with what might be in it. I was freaked out. But I was not about to give up with all those other people heading farther out to deeper, darker water. My arms felt like lead. I was not in the kind of shape in which I needed to be. It put a fine point on what I needed to do to get ready. I started swimming with much more focus and determination. I kept at it with the weekend group and became more comfortable and even moderately relaxed during those ocean swims.

This was northern California on the Pacific Ocean. I was in a wetsuit, the water was very cold, the waves were big, and the salt water got in my mouth. Sound fun? Not at first. But once I got past all of that, the feeling of freedom was irresistible. No constraints. No walls. No turns and no counting lengths. Big, wide, open expanses in all directions. Just nature. I have always viewed open water ocean swimming as a bit of a test. The swimmer has to overcome the waves, the currents, and his fear. While there are no lane lines or pool walls to close them in, there is also no resting at the end of the pool. Navigation is always tricky and vitally important. If the swimmer is not careful to frequently sight ahead on a target, it is easy to get off course. My morning swim group enjoyed these challenging conditions, and soon I joined in their enthusiasm wholeheartedly. Ocean swimming was new to me and I was getting good at it. Once again—and critically important—I was getting good at something with no "considering."

The old PA students' group that had been with us on our prenuptial honeymoon continued to vacation together frequently. We all had kids. We had three; Eric and Cristin had two; and Pat and Susan had one. In the main room of the ski cabin we rented one year was a bevy of rollaway cots. I wore my prized Telluride sweatpants. They were extra special because we had had great difficulty finding sweatpants with the Telluride logo down the left leg. (A logo on the right leg would be useless, as it would be cut off.) I was walking through the room on crutches, navigating my foot and crutch placement carefully to miss beds, ski clothes, and people's feet. As I passed near Susan, without me knowing it, she was in the midst of a profound debate with herself. *If he was me and I was him, he would trip me for sure. If I don't trip him, I'm catering to the disability and that is a sure no-no. So should I do it or not?* She had to decide quickly. Out went her foot and she got me good. Without all the obstacles, I would have just done a stumble, hop, hop, and recovered. But one crutch caught on a bed, the other caught on a ski boot, and I went down hard. As I went down, everyone else in the room looked aghast at Susan. They all thought, *How could you do that, Susan? You just tripped a guy on crutches.* She was pretty upset with herself, thinking this is not what she intended to have happen.

The worst of it was that one of the bed frames got a good hold of the pant leg right by the Telluride logo and ripped it up the whole leg. When I came up, there was no blood, no pain, but there were ruined sweatpants. Susan was still in shock. For the ripped sweatpants, and only for that, Susan was in trouble with me. She was buying me new, logo-on-the-left-leg Telluride sweatpants or else.

To people who knew me, there was no issue with tripping me or challenging me in ways no different from anyone else. In some ways, people who knew me well gave me even less leeway than others. I have made my athletic life highly visible to others, so people have gotten used to my accomplishments. And because I have accomplished so much, they do not realize how difficult it is and how hard I continue to have to work.

Every father of small children has a "close call" story of survival of one of his kids. But not many involve a naked, one-legged rescue. We were visiting good friends who had an outdoor pool. Naturally, the kids wanted to get in right away when we got there, no delay. The other fathers and I agreed to change into our suits out by the side of the pool while the ladies went inside to change more discretely. At two and a half, Zac was competent with his water wings. At nine, Brendan was a fish in the water and was down at the deep end. However, Joanna, who was only eighteen months and still new to walking, was not swimming at all yet. I was in a chair by the end where Joanna was. I had my pants off and my suit just starting to come on my leg when I watched in horror as she blithely stepped down that fateful last step right into water over her head. I didn't think; I just leaped. I might have made a clean rescue if not for a large riding toy between my chair and the water's edge that caught on my dangling bathing suit. That slowed my body down just enough that my leap failed to clear the edge of the pool, and so my leg came down on the concrete edge. The suit that had caused this ignominious water entry was innocently hanging back on the kids' riding toy. But I still reached Joanna and, with a quick swipe, had her back above water. She had not even had time to take a breath underwater. In fact she was laughing. She wasn't the only one. Just then, the women arrived to find me in a sorry state of undress with a hematoma on my shin rapidly growing to the size of a tennis ball. Since Joanna was fine—still happy and oblivious not only to her close call, but to why Daddy was making Mommy laugh so hard—the ladies had quite a laugh at my expense as I struggled to get my suit back on.

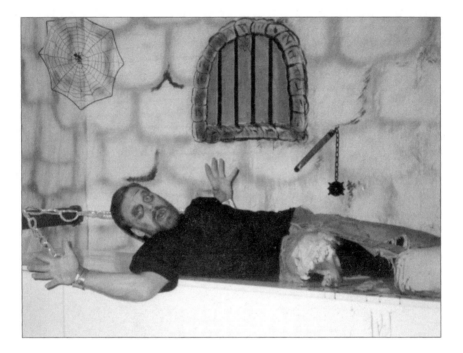

EIGHT

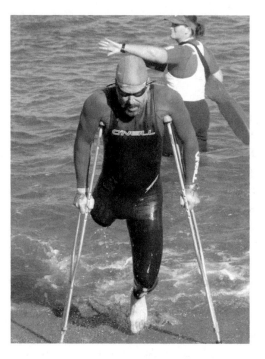

SWIMMING THROUGH SHARKS

I'm convinced that about half of what separates the successful entrepreneurs from the non-successful ones is pure perseverance.

—Steve Jobs, entrepreneur, innovator

The most essential factor is persistence—the determination never to allow your energy or enthusiasm to be dampened by the discouragement that must inevitably come.

—James Whitcomb Riley, poet

Our greatest weakness lies in giving up. The most certain way to succeed is always to try just one more time.

— Thomas Alva Edison, inventor

I became hooked on a weekly ocean swim every Friday morning before work. Along with my swim partner Steve, we went to Cowell Beach in downtown Santa Cruz right around sunrise. We swam fifty-two weeks a year except after a big rainstorm, when the runoff made the water too polluted.

In the winter, when the air temperature was forty-five to fifty degrees and the water temperature was at its lowest of the year, at around fifty-two, it was especially challenging. When we got out of the water, already close to hypothermic, the air and wind blowing on our wet skin and wetsuits cooled us down fast. We raced to retrieve our keys out from their hiding places and unlock the car before our fingers got so cold they couldn't work the locks. We turned the heat in our cars to full blast. Then we had to clean off in outdoor, cold-water showers designed for surfers to rinse off sand. We did that fast, too, and jumped back into the car. No matter what we did, we started to develop a deep shiver. I mean a really deep shiver that shakes your whole body and lasts about thirty minutes. The server at the Peet's Coffee shop must have thought we had a neurological condition because we asked for our coffee, shaking uncontrollably, and then held the coffee cup in both hands, still shaking as we put it up to our mouths.

Steve kept tabs on upcoming swimming and triathlon events. They were going to hold an annual swim from Alcatraz Island back to San Francisco, landing at Aquatic Park near the famous Ghirardelli sign.

"We should do it," he said. "The distance is only 1.5 miles and only the Anglin Brothers and Frank Lee Morris were rumored to have finished the swim. Their bodies were never found."

Huge ships pass back and forth where we'd be swimming. What no one can see is the fast current that wants to take the itinerant swimmer to an even scarier place: out under the Golden Gate Bridge—where there *are* man-eating sharks.

This was a grand and intimidating challenge. The whole point of Alcatraz as a prison was that it was impossible to escape. In subsequent years, this swim would come to be considered the granddaddy of all open water swims. I wanted to do it. It intimidated everyone, so my doing it would be quite an accomplishment. I would have to work very hard to get ready. Just thinking about it months in advance gave me butterflies.

To get ready, we increased the frequency of our swims off the wharf in Santa Cruz to twice a week. Our usual Friday morning swim out to the end of the wharf was just shy of a mile. To lengthen the course, we followed the swim buoys put out by the lifeguards. The buoys demarcate a dividing line between a swimming area and a surfing area. The surfing area is the famed Steamers Lane of legendary surfing. Swimming out along this buoy line left the swimmers pretty exposed. Occasionally that was a problem. One day we saw the fog bank way out on the horizon, yet close in it was crystal clear. We swam out to the end of the buoy line when, all of a sudden, the fog swept in and engulfed us. We could not see more than four feet. Steve thought the way back in was one way and I thought it was another. If we were wrong, we could be swimming until we hit Japan. Since I tend to have a better instinct for directions, Steve went with my gut and we headed my way. We finally found the pilings of the wharf, which meant I was "only" off by ninety degrees. At least we were able to follow the wharf pilings toward the shore safely. After that, we got special waterproof strobe lights to wear on our arms. We also carried waterproof whistles. People who knew we were doing this started calling us "geek swimmers." We focused seriously on safety. We even practiced towing each other to shore as if the drag-ee was out cold.

Each morning of a swim, Steve and I met in the deserted parking lot right about—or sometimes before—dawn. The sun rises over the water in Santa Cruz. It is counterintuitive, but Santa Cruz sits on the northern tip of Monterey Bay, making east to your left as you look south across the bay. It was quiet, lonely, and dramatic as the light first appeared in the sky. The water in which we were about to immerse ourselves was dark and cold. Challenging ourselves in this way made me feel strong and resolute. We'd quietly change into our wetsuits, put on double caps for warmth, strap our safety lights and whistles to our upper arms, and put on goggles. I would add fins and a nose plug. At the water's edge, Steve went through a process to prepare himself for the cold water I liked to call his "chicken dance." He dipped a toe in the water and then hopped around. Then he got in up to his ankles and hopped around. Then his waist. Meanwhile, I had my flipper, goggles, and nose plug on—ready to go. While waiting for him to finish his dance, I sat on the sand just above the wave line where I would leave my crutches. After Steve had taken a few strokes and his breathing was under control, he'd look back at me and wave. That was my signal to head in. With my flipper on, I hopped backwards down the beach and into the water.

The breaking waves were a balance challenge. I forged ahead (or should I say, behind?), hopping backwards quickly deeper and deeper while withstanding the increasing force of the breaking waves against my solitary leg. I could not look down because, if I did, I would be looking at moving water, which would disrupt my balance. Just as a wave was about to hit me high enough to reach my waist, I turned and dove into that wave and started stroking. I always let out a massive gasp as the super cold water hit my upper body, but I found the best thing was to immediately stroke very hard to generate my own heat. We used wetsuits with no arms to prevent our strokes from being hindered, which meant our bare arms got quite cold. Sometimes when the water temperature was in the low fifties, first exposure resulted in an ice cream headache. That, too, faded with hard swimming.

Steve's water entry ritual was all a process to help him avoid cold water and exercise-induced asthma. However, before Steve became an Ironman triathlete, his ritual didn't completely work and he was not able to immediately start stroking all out as I was. At first, he would lag behind, but he would keep at it and soon be cranking at full steam. By halfway out to the end of the wharf, Steve always started to pull in front of me. Our strokes were smooth and strong by now. Not only did we no longer feel the cold, but also we actually felt quite comfortable. It seemed our muscles and joints worked better in the cold. That or we were just too numb to feel any pain they might be having. The cold and the buoyancy provided by the salt water and wetsuits improved our efficiency; we swam faster and used less energy than in warm water pools.

At the end of the wharf that sticks one half mile straight out into the bay from Cowell Cove Beach, we were right next to the sea lions' hangout. Reaching that wharf was a spectacular moment of peace and quiet. Swimming in open water is one of the most liberating things I ever get to do. The feeling of freedom is so strong and so compelling; it overwhelms any feeling of discomfort from the cold or the fear. It is the closest thing to a religious experience I've ever had.

I have to admit we showed pretty poor judgment once when the NOAA (National Oceanic and Atmospheric Administration) data from the Mile Buoy was showing thirteen-foot swells every seven seconds. Mile Buoy is a half-mile farther out in Monterey Bay than the end of the wharf. Getting out in those conditions was extremely difficult, and the swim felt like a rollercoaster. We saw swells actually touch the decking on the Santa Cruz Wharf, twenty-two feet above high tide. Had you been standing at the end of the wharf, the swells would have reached your feet. Swimming out, one wave did push Steve to the ocean floor hard and shot him out of the water like a missile. One of us thought that was funny (and it wasn't Steve). Just beyond the breaking waves, I ran into some kelp. I stopped because it was all over my face. Steve was swimming right next to me at the time. While stopped, I parted the kelp in front of my face like a wig and said, "Look, I'm Whoopi Goldberg." That time, both of us were laughing as we bobbed up and down like corks on the big swells.

Thirteen-foot walls of water could have easily snapped our necks when heading back to the beach. Because the backwash was so strong, it worked against us pulling us back in as we tried to get up the beach, and we withstood several poundings before we finally made it out of the water. We timed it like surfers and fought to get as far up on the sand as possible to avoid being pulled back in. It was frightening, and we vowed to be more cautious about wave size from then on.

We did a couple of events prior to taking the Alcatraz plunge. In Santa Cruz every summer, they hold the Rough Water Swim.

This is a one-mile, all-out sprint from the Santa Cruz Main Beach on the east side of the wharf, out to the end, and back to land on the west side at Cowell Beach. We used to joke that to give me a little edge, we should take the discarded right leg that had been cut off from my wetsuit and stuff it full of newspaper. Then, while all the swimmers were congregating at the water's edge, we would throw the stuffed leg out into the surf. In my imagination, it would drift around for a bit until someone noticed it and let out a terrified scream. Okay, it would have been a sick thing to do, but it sure would have been funny.

The day finally arrived for our first attempt at Alcatraz. I couldn't sleep for two nights before the swim. The morning of the event, we left Santa Cruz at 4:30 a.m. We had to be at water's edge by 6:30, and we were taking no chances. Steve never took chances. When Steve locked his car, which reliably auto-locked all the doors with the push of one button, he walked around to check every door. When he used a remote to close his garage door, he patiently waited until it settled in the down position and showed no sign of spontaneously popping back up, even though it never had. Steve packed every single shirt, pair of pants, and underwear each in its very own separate Ziploc bag before putting it into his suitcase. He brought a large thermos filled with hot water to make for a more comfortable warm water rinse after a swim. He kept his cell phone in its own Tupperware container. "It protects it," he told me when I challenged this practice as unusual. A bit obsessive, yes, but you need some form of crazy to swim in such rough, cold, open waters. Who was I to criticize his version?

Nine hundred swimmers congregated in predawn hours at the San Francisco Maritime Museum for the inaugural Alcatraz Sharkfest swim. After registration, we all donned our wetsuits. I had to pee every ten minutes from non-stop nerves. Finally, when everyone was organized, we formed a procession and walked the five or six blocks down to the red and white ferry line terminal at Fisherman's Wharf. I, of course, walked on crutches carrying my goggles and fin. Naturally, I got a few stares. I kept glancing furtively to my left. There it was, out in the middle of a cold, rough bay: Alcatraz Island, shrouded in mist, looking ominous and very far away.

Everyone loaded up on the commuter ferryboat and we rode out to the island. Steve and I got up on the top deck so we could see all the angles and plot our course. The city grew farther and farther away. Everyone tried to study landmarks. Navigation in this sort of swim is everything, and it is vastly more difficult than one would think. Just two inches of water in front of your face while swimming will block your eyes entirely, and there are certainly waves much bigger than two inches in the San Francisco Bay. The ferry stopped one hundred feet off the National Park dock on the south side of the island, the side facing the Oakland Bay Bridge. The doors of the boat faced directly toward the Golden Gate Bridge, ensconced in fog. Everyone jumped out the big double doors. It was eight feet down to the water, as this boat normally docked at a high wharf where people in business clothes loaded and unloaded for their workday commute. I went first so someone could grab the crutches and get them out of people's way. The crew agreed to take the crutches back to the finish area and hand them to me as I got out of the water.

It took fifteen or more minutes for all nine hundred swimmers to empty the ferryboat. That meant the first one in (me, immediately followed by Steve) had to tread water all that time. The water temperature was no big deal; it was actually a few degrees warmer than Santa Cruz water in January. The starting line was made up of all the kayaks, paddleboards, and rubber runabouts that formed our chaperone flotilla. Steve and I agreed on a strategy: we would get to an edge of the crowd, as opposed to dead center, so we wouldn't be kicked to death when the swim started.

The start signal was the horn on the ferry. We were off. It was incredibly hard to navigate that swim not only because of the rough water, but also because of the sideways current. There was a current even though they tried to time the start to be at slack high tide. The current never stops, partly because the final surge of the Sacramento River, coming across the central valley down from the Sierras, splits around Alcatraz on its way out under the Golden Gate Bridge.

I felt tired. My arms felt like lead, but I think it was mental not physical. I thought I was prepared, but I needed to prepare even harder. I got mouthfuls of saltwater from the waves. Progress across the bay seemed snail slow. It was nothing like swimming in the pool. To counteract the waves, I slowed down my stroke to make it longer and stronger. I turned my head farther to get a breath and looked up every dozen or so strokes to sight where I was trying to go. The huge crowd we started with seemed to have thinned out to the point where I saw almost no one—including Steve. *Was I being left in the dust?* We were separated quite early and I never saw him again until the finish.

As I swam across the stretch from Alcatraz Island to the break-water that forms Aquatic Park, the strong current moved me inexorably toward the Golden Gate Bridge. I didn't sense it at all, as the entire mass of water in which I was swimming was moving en masse. As I neared the breakwater, the current actually acceler-ated, as the mass of water pushed up against the cement wall and had nowhere else to go but out the bay. On strong current years, the narrow opening of the breakwater entrance to Aquatic Park, and the finish line, has a very strong current passing in front of it, and swimmers have to fight hard just to get through the opening. Weak swimmers navigating too close to the downstream side can get pushed right past the opening and require a boat to assist them back upstream. Others get pushed into the wooden pilings and scraped up. Many swimmers finish with blood on their legs and arms. Even strong swimmers have to point themselves at forty-five degrees to the opening and bear down, sprinting to get through the rushing current. There is a moment of panic as you think you aren't moving despite swimming at all-out anaerobic capacity, and still you can see the huge pier on your right getting slightly closer as the current pushes you. On top of the pier, people scream things we cannot hear—probably helpful advice like, "Swim like hell!" or "Hey do you realize you are about to get smashed into this pier I am standing on?"

I came in upstream of the opening to Aquatic Park. Good thing, because the flow can be as fast as six miles per hour toward the Golden Gate Bridge. A fast swimmer can hold two miles per hour, so if I had gotten downstream of the opening, I wouldn't have been able to beat the current back up to make it through. I'd have had the ignominious experience of being picked up by a runabout boat, hauled upstream, and dropped off to try again. Everyone would know if that happened.

I made it through the opening between the breakwaters that define Aquatic Park and started the last leg in the flat water toward the beach. Seeing a huge crowd at the finish took away the leaden feeling in my arms and I cranked away. Steve was ahead of me somewhere. I made it to the finish and saw Steve with my crutches come racing back into the water to hand them to me. I was still in waist-deep water, so I could stand up with crutches. I could tell the crowd was trying to figure out what was going on. They started yelling for me to get up and run to the finish line like all the other people who came in. When I moved far enough out of the water for them to see why I needed crutches, they let out a deafening roar and broke into raucous cheering. I had never experienced a crowd of people cheering for me. It was a fantastic feeling.

This swim is officially called the Alcatraz Sharkfest, and their logo is a huge great white shark. Everyone assumes there are sharks in San Francisco Bay, which made Alcatraz such an ideal location for a prison. However, inside the bay, the only sharks are small, bottom-feeding scavenger sharks that do not bother people. Nearby, outside the Golden Gate in the area called the Farallons, there certainly are great whites—lots of them—and they do occasionally attack surfers.

To a shark, the sight from below nine hundred people with 1,799 legs thrashing must be very intimidating and not at all appetizing. If they were going to go after one of those morsels, Steve and I always said they would work at the edges first, so we never stayed near the edge. Furthermore, as I was fond of saying, if one did see me, he'd think, *someone's already working on him so I'll leave him be.*

At 1.5 miles as the crow flies, the Alcatraz event is not the longest. But the water is rough, cold, and intimidating, and right next to the Golden Gate Bridge. That's what makes it breathtaking and elite, as well as addictive. I go back every year and surprisingly—since I am not getting any younger—I keep getting faster. It's never the same swim twice.

People completely ignore my "situation" when doing this swim. In fact, new swimmers assume they will not be as fast as I am. Think about that. This is what someone with a disability dreams of. Far from "good considering," people instead inquire about my best time and what my goal is next year. People ask my advice on the swim because I am one of the more experienced swimmers. Spectators who come to the swim know they would not be able to do it. I have created the ideal scenario for an event that, in spite of a disability, I can do and most cannot. This combination is a critical element in maintaining the self-esteem I need in the face of constant and ongoing challenges.

To prepare for this swim, I must work harder than my two-legged compatriots. I'm used to this. It's true about anything I determine to do well. For the swim, I am in the pool swimming, increasing the length of my workouts for months leading up to the event. I maintain a steady state of about ten thousand yards (almost six miles) per week all year round. If I don't stick to this regimen, I slip backwards quickly. Building back up is unpleasant and time-consuming, probably largely due to my diminished lung capacity, which is taxed by distance swimming. As the Alcatraz date approaches, which is always during the summer, I switch from indoor pool swimming to mostly outdoor open water swimming. In California that was ocean swimming, and in Boston it is Walden Pond (of Henry David Thoreau fame) swimming.

Every year, I still get butterflies before the swim, but after more than a dozen times, I can focus more on the event and make it even more fun. I know how to prepare. I know how to navigate it. And my times have been dropping. Every year, I finish in the top dozen for my age group, and it is mostly younger people who beat me. Perhaps now it is okay to say, "He's fast considering . . . he's getting old!"

As I began to understand what the roar of the crowd meant as I got out of the water, I began learning to use my situation to impact people in a positive way. I turned this swim event into a vehicle for charity fundraising for the Boston Healthcare for the Homeless Program, where Carole works. It's a great cause, and people get excited when someone does something that they can't do, especially when its leveraged to help a good charity.

What the whitewater rafting through Freight Train, the one-footed barefoot waterskiing, the swimming across San Francisco Bay, and all the athletics taught me was that I could tackle really difficult things and succeed. It finally dawned on me: if I could do those things, I could do anything. I was thriving. I had overcome the loss of a limb, the loss of a lung, the loss of assurance that I would live. If I could deal with all of that, I could deal with other equally difficult challenges, like starting a company. Getting an idea, building a team, getting it funded, taking a product to market. I knew these were among the hardest things to do in my industry, but as a result of my athletic successes, I had the self-confidence to give it a try.

I had worked at Borland for five years. It was an important phase of my career, filled with both good and bad lessons. I became a very strong manager with a high human resource aptitude strongly instilled in me by Borland's outstanding approach to hiring, firing, compensation, motivation, and even layoffs. There were many big challenges during the Borland years. Microsoft was responsible for many of them. I ran one product, *Borland C++*, that was maintaining a bigger market share than Microsoft. And they were determined to change that no matter how out of line—or frankly illegal—their methods. Quietly, Microsoft's treatment of Netscape in the browser wars was being scrutinized by the authorities, and storm clouds were beginning to form around whether Microsoft was acting as an illegal monopoly. Ultimately, I ended up on the front lines in that battle and the Department of Justice deposed me twice to garner critical evidence that ultimately helped find Microsoft guilty of acting illegally.

One last bold move was left in Borland, and I was to be a central part of that. Borland acquired a startup company called Open Environment in Boston that would be central to their strategy to get back out in front. I was the one chosen to go to Boston and integrate this startup into the parent company and product line. It was to be a one-year assignment, and I tried to get the family to look at it as an adventure. We figured we could put up with anything for a year. Carole wouldn't work that year, as Borland agreed to pay her salary while she took a leave of absence. We cashed in some stock options and started a total remodel of our house in California. We planned to strip the first floor down to the studs and move the kitchen from one end of the house to the other, while adding solid cherry custom built-in cabinets. All this would amount to $140,000 and could be done while we lived in a rental home in Boston.

We picked the New England town that our research showed had some of the best schools in the area: Newton, Massachusetts. We found a rental home and enrolled the kids in school. We quickly got a large dose of the sad state of the California schools compared to Massachusetts. Newton schools still had art and music, school buses, foreign language, a full compliment of sports, and a rich after-school program, all of which had been victims of Proposition 13 in California. Massachusetts's schools remained well funded and ranked near the top in the country. Academically, the kids were a year behind their Massachusetts peers in science and math—a year they would luckily quickly make up. By October, as Carole and I left our first back-to-school night event, we knew we could not leave these schools. If we moved back to California before the kids were done with school, Carole and I agreed, we would be horrible parents.

In early fall, when Borland missed its revenue target for the quarter and the board immediately fired the CEO, I had been in Boston for only three months. That CEO had been instrumental in my support structure back at the company, as had been his second in command, my good friend and boss, Paul Gross. Paul received a very lucrative offer from Microsoft and took it. This was after they had given other huge offers to key engineers throughout Borland by renting out the hotel across the street and posting flyers at the company to come across the street and get the "offer of a lifetime." That was later declared an illegal hiring practice, but only after it was too late. Paul got a million dollar sign-on bonus, tons of stock options, and a huge salary. Money is an amazing motivator, so all his many years of animus towards Microsoft were quickly forgotten. He had begged me to go to Boston, saying I would be holding the crown jewels of the company, only to abandon ship three months later, leaving me trying to hold the fort from three thousand miles away. Now my only two lifelines to the parent company were gone and, as is always the case, when the mother ship is going down, those in the outpost get major whiplash.

A small group of people at the acquired company in Boston came to me with an idea for a new company and asked me to join them. I continued to be a risk-taker in most, if not all, aspects of life, and so I said "yes." I even named the new venture while sitting at one of Zac's soccer games. We would call it "Net Propulsion" because it would, in some ways, speed up the Web. I was now on a path to learn how the world of startups worked, including how to raise money from venture capitalists. No longer just a sports risk-taker, I was now also a business risk-taker and well on my way to becoming a true entrepreneur.

We needed outside investors to fund our idea, so we began to pitch it to local venture capitalists. The idea for our new company was well received and we got several Venture Capitalists (VCs) interested. Along the way one gave me the feedback I had been expecting, but dreading, to hear: I was not what they had in mind for CEO. I was not ready. Although I had set my sights on becoming a CEO, I must admit that I, too, didn't feel I was quite ready. Still, I was the oldest and most experienced member of our group. I had been their boss at Borland, so leading the company seemed the only option even to them. The VCs, however, saw what was obvious: I had no sales background. All of this strongly resonated with my own self-perception that I was not qualified to be CEO, at least not yet. I wanted to become CEO because it was the hardest job in business to attain, and I was driven to attain it in the same way I reacted to any stiff challenge. But it wasn't to be then; I needed more CEO training. I took the VCs' advice and agreed that I would not be in an operating role at this startup and would instead just act as an advisor. Because I was determined to become a CEO eventually, I decided to go get that training somewhere else as opposed to taking a vice president role at Net Propulsion.

When we finally got a term sheet from an interested VC, the decision that I was going elsewhere was already a done deal in my mind. But Ted, the new VC, decided I was the guy he wanted as CEO. He begged me to reconsider. However, by voicing the doubts I felt, the earlier VC, who was not investing in this deal, had convinced me; I was not ready, and forcing myself into that role could hurt Net Propulsion's chances for success. As I look back with many years of experience, both as CEO and as non-CEO in five more startups, I see how wrong the first VC was and how right Ted was. The initial founder CEO is usually not the one that takes the company into the realm of high-volume sales and profitability. The early CEO is more often the guy who understands the technology intimately and can articulate what it is and why it is needed. That, I know now, was an apt description of me, but at the time, I knew nothing about starting a company from scratch and was easily influenced by a VC playing into my own self-doubts.

I secured the funding for Net Propulsion (whose name was shortly changed to Webspective), and then I became an advisor to them and not an employee. I went back to the VCs I had liked best to ask for advice. "Which of your portfolio companies should I join to fill in the gaps in my study to become CEO?" I asked. Paul, one of the VCs we had pitched to, said I should join one of his portfolio companies where the CEO was a consummate sales guy so I could learn that aspect of business from him. He gave me two choices and a little push toward the one that, as it turned out, was in the most trouble and needed fixing. Paul needed someone like me to join the struggling company as CTO because he counted on me to help save his investment.

I joined ten-year-old Novasoft, which was fourth place in a market that was in overall decline. The CEO was a fireball of energy who had been VP of Sales at his last company where he had gotten rich. He had also made the VCs of his last company rich, and so he convinced the VCs he could be CEO (a common pattern). The VCs then convinced me that I would learn to be CEO best from him. I was naive beyond belief.

Just eight months into the job, the VCs staged a dinner with me. Meeting in the evening like this—at a restaurant—was not how they had done things in the past. My guard was up. Sure enough, the minute we met at the restaurant, it was clear the meeting was about the CEO. The investors wanted to find out if the management team had lost faith in the CEO. It turned out that everyone had lost confidence in him, and now with the board against him too, it was over.

We had quickly gone from "Go here and learn to be CEO," to "Sorry. Learning is over. We want you to be CEO now."

I said, "No, how could I possibly be ready so quickly?"

They said, "If your answer is no, then we are prepared to shut down the company. Either you accept the CEO role or we fire everyone tomorrow."

It was a King Solomon's cut-the-baby-in-half choice: I either become CEO way before I was ready or we shut down the company.

Seventy-five employees, dozens of customers, and more than $30 million of venture capital invested to date would all go down the drain. I reluctantly agreed.

There I was, a first-time CEO with the new VP of Sales the previous CEO had just hired thinking he was more qualified for the job, a users' conference with hundreds of customers attending in a month, a company that would run out of cash in two months, and an overall business that was declining. Can you say stress? Job one was to raise money and fast, which I had no experience doing. This would be the company's round F of VC money. Most VCs stop putting more money in at round C.

The company was burning way too much cash and struggling in a moribund market. I had to cut expenses, and that meant painful layoffs of almost half the company. Furthermore, I quickly needed to move the company into a new market while leveraging its current talent base and technology. Unbelievably frightening. Unbelievably stressful. I tried to remember that these challenges were nothing compared to the death threat I received when I was nineteen. This was how I always put a difficult situation into perspective, no matter how dire. Nevertheless, I still woke up with cold sweats many nights, especially when my actions affected other people, their livelihood, and their families. I never inured to firing or laying people off.

I survived running the user's conference, but barely. I survived the raising of the next round of VC financing, but barely. I settled down to focus on learning how to be CEO and running the company. At first, this was an extension of what I had been doing as CTO, but it became obvious to me and my senior team that maintaining current course and speed would mean disaster—and quite soon. We were in a shrinking market, which is bad enough for the market leader, but for the number four player it is certain death. We had to get out of the document management market and fast. We had to find a way to use our current assets (people, investors, technology) to get into a new market that had growth potential—one in which we could somehow become dominant. This is a textbook statement for what startups have to do all the time when their best laid plans don't work out. I liked to call it "bobbing and weaving."

In the spirit of bobbing and weaving our way out of a dying market, I worked hard to reshape the company into something completely new and different. The new idea actually came from Carole. In her job treating patients with AIDS, as she had in Santa Cruz, Carole was starting to use the Internet. Rapid changes were occurring in the treatment of AIDS that meant life over death, but those treatments were still six months away from publication in traditional refereed print publications. She wanted to use the web to access the latest, up-to-the-minute AIDS treatments. Sitting next to me one evening while she was online, Carole exclaimed that she thought what she was reading was quack medicine.

I asked, "Well, where did you find that?"

"From AltaVista," she said.

"But AltaVista is just a search engine," I explained. "Where did AltaVista get it from?"

"It's a no-name site."

"Well then you may not want to trust it, especially for life and death treatments you might use tomorrow," I said. "You can't trust it if you don't know them and can't vouch for them."

"So where should I go then?" Carole asked.

"To a reputable site."

"Okay, so if I go to MedScape [a well known medical site] can I trust their content?"

"Actually, that's not guaranteed," I reluctantly said. "Because it's so easy to make you think it's MedScape when really it's not."

"Then this web is useless," she said in disgust turning off her computer. "Someone could die if I have to wait to get this information in print, and someone could die if I get bogus information. This web thing is useless. So when are you going to fix it?"

That's it, I thought. The new direction for the company would be enabling users to tell whether the content they were looking at in a browser was bona fide and therefore trustworthy.

With the new idea, we changed the name of the company to Factpoint and set off in the new direction. But time was running out for us as the investors have a time limit on their funds and this company was already eight years old. The investors impatiently asked me to find a fresh investor or to sell the company. At the 1999 Halloween board meeting, we presented four choices to the board;

finding a new investor (which had not worked so far), selling the company (which also had not worked), getting a modest additional investment from existing investors (which we all felt sure they would go for), and for completeness, shutting down the company. Unbelievably, they picked option number four, shutting Factpoint down. That meant firing all forty-five employees, including myself, the next morning. With our new name and direction, we had found some initial traction with a few impressive customers in the new market. But the time limit on the investors' funds trumped this progress and we had to give it up.

I left the Halloween board meeting with real tears in my eyes for what I had to do next. The next morning, the fired employees were surprised, angry, and scared to so suddenly have it all end.

I still believed in the new direction we had started to take. I asked the investors if I could buy the intellectual property from them. They offered it to me for one million dollars. At first, I thought that was reasonable, so I began to talk to new VCs about funding a brand new company that would start with the one million dollars of new technology and the patents we had filed on it. But when I heard one of the investors in the shut down venture suggest that perhaps that was not enough money for the assets because, he speculated, maybe I had a buyer on the side and was going to quickly "flip" that technology for a lot more than one million, I quickly withdrew my offer. There was no trust. They wanted to assume the worst. So I thought of another way. I went to the lawyers tasked with the liquidation of all the company's assets and asked them for what amount they thought I could buy that same intellectual property in the liquidation process. They said $65,000 would get it, and all I had to do was wait the prescribed amount of time to make sure there were no higher competing bids. It was with this $65,000 intellectual property that, with a good friend, Dave Chen, I started WorldCert, which was sold seven years later for $125 million.

I would be COO this time and Dave would be CEO. The company was bi-coastal between Boston and Portland, Oregon. I would do most of the traveling. Every other week for eighteen months, I flew to Portland. (Nope, I never do things the easy way.)

Dave had agreed to be WorldCert CEO for only eighteen months, and so when we reached that milestone it was time for me to step up. But the company was not in good shape. We had overspent and overbuilt. Worse, the technology was not ready for the market. It needed my technical full-time attention. In addition, we had no sales, so sales and marketing needed my full-time attention, too. What we really needed was a CEO from the outside who had strong sales and marketing instincts with whom I could collaborate and split all these jobs. I needed to focus on fixing our technology while he focused on sales and marketing. I found someone I thought would be a perfect fit with me, and Dave agreed. The proposed CEO was a business partner at a company with whom we had done a lot of work. He was thrilled. He had already prepared his own business plan to start a company, and this gave him a platform that was much further along. It was to be his first time as CEO.

Our new CEO had great business instincts and figured out a good way to get us revenue quickly on a business model that was simple and proven: sell security to web sites that accept credit cards over the web so people's credit card numbers stayed safe and secure. He went back to the division of the company where he used to work and offered to buy that little division outright. Because they knew him, they were willing to make a very sweet deal. It was a brilliant move that gave us a way to get revenue fast and is the reason the company survived.

The new CEO was taking charge of the company and moving it in a new direction with strong support of the new VC we had brought in. This new direction would ultimately be hugely successful, and five years later he was able to sell the little company Dave and I had started with $65,000 for more than $100 million. But as frequently happens, his vision for the company and mine diverged. He was the CEO that I had chosen, so it was time for me to go. While these departures of the founder might not be uncommon, they are very painful to live through. It feels like you are being torn from "your baby."

After swimming the Alcatraz Sharkfest a dozen times, it finally struck me: I was swimming through harmless sharks in San Francisco Bay once a year, but I was swimming through business sharks every day in my startup companies. The latter were proving to be quite dangerous.

NINE

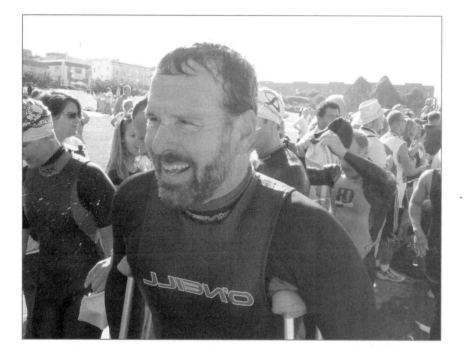

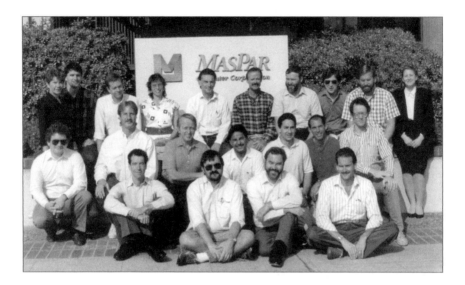

INCORRIGIBLE ENTREPRENEUR

If a child shows himself to be incorrigible, he should be decently and quietly beheaded at the age of twelve, lest he grow to maturity, marry, and perpetuate his kind.

—Don Marquis, US humorist

Entrepreneurs are simply those who understand that there is little difference between obstacle and opportunity and are able to turn both to their advantage.

— Niccolo Machiavelli, political philosopher

Why did I keep doing venture capitalist-backed startups when they were so painful? Webspective was my first, and the VCs there told me I was not ready to be CEO. Novasoft was my second, and when they decided to fire the CEO, they suddenly flip-flopped and said I was ready, only to have the company shut down for taking too long to turn around. At WorldCert, the CEO I hired to come join me as a partner had a different vision for the company strongly backed by the newest VC we brought in so I had to depart. Why did I keep going back for more? Well, for one thing, two of those startups had indeed been bought by much bigger companies and made the investors and the employees (including me) a fair bit of money, validating all our initial ideas and hard work. But money was never my major motivator; my primary driving force was the challenge and thrill of creating a new company from nothing but my ideas.

In my forties, I had finally reached a balance where I could separate what I had been through with cancer—chemotherapy, being told I had zero chance of survival, and all the challenges that come from living with a disability—from my career. However, as with all other aspects of my life, in my career I was inexorably drawn to those things that others considered an almost unachievable challenge. I refused to fail, and so when a startup ended badly, I instinctively picked myself up time after time and tried again. It was like falling my first time skiing one-legged. It hurt a lot, but if I didn't get up and try again, I would never get it right.

To a certain extent, I fell into being a serial entrepreneur in much the same way I fell into finishing college, getting my PhD, and joining my first startup in California. The opportunity was right in front of me, it sounded good, the thrill was there, and most of all, there didn't seem to be anything better to do at the moment.

To be able to fall into a pattern of entrepreneur-hood, I had to have a high dose of one critical ingredient: optimism. Incorrigible entrepreneurs are first and foremost incorrigible optimists. This has to be true because almost everything is stacked against them from day one. If the slightest thing goes haywire with the team, the investors, the market, the product, the competition, the customers, the economy, and who-knows-what-else, it's game over for a startup in its fragile early days.

Why was I an optimist? I had as good a reason as anybody not to be. But I'm not sure you get to choose. Maybe it's in your DNA. I started my career as a programmer and, as most computer scientists agree, that weeds out non-optimists. Optimism sure is a useful thing when you are being buffeted by one challenge after another. My particular brand of optimism was really a constant need to look forward. I always looked forward to the next meal, the next trip, the next date, the next meeting. As I lay flat on my back in a hospital, the future did not look very good, yet I still tried to imagine walking, skiing—being normal somehow. When the present is tough, imagining a better future and moving to make it happen is an act of self-preservation. The harder things got, the more I focused on a better future and set out to make my dreams a reality with hard work and perseverance. This ability to focus became inculcated in my core being, and it was in full operation in all aspects of my life. It looked, tasted, and felt like optimism, and it worked to keep me going in the face of huge adversity in the world of high-tech startups.

My first startup began in California in 1988. By 2009, I had been intimately involved with a total of ten. What they all had in common had indeed become infectious and addictive. The teams were small and tight. Everyone was aligned behind the same goals. We were all in it together like paddlers in a raft in Class V rapids, depending on each other for survival. Everyone took the same risk and had the same potential for reward if we "survived." Since people are not exactly coerced into joining startups, you end up with a team of people who share many basic likes and dislikes, as well as important aspects of their personalities. This makes for a more cohesive, bonded group. People at startups are self-selected to work very hard.

In each startup, and for at least its first year, the close-knit team had insatiable energy and unstoppable drive aiming toward the goal. The goal was always the same at first: get a product ready for market and then find the first few customers who needed it and would pay for it. This made getting everyone to focus quite natural at first. That becomes much harder to do later when lots of different customers want different things, when competitors from all different directions begin to buffet the company's little boat, and when the company starts to grow and hire people who are not of the same ilk the boat starts to take on some water.

During the very early days of a startup, in spite of working long, hard hours—or perhaps because of it—the teams are ready to celebrate the tiniest little victories. The product showed its first sign of life? Celebrate. Had a first meeting with a customer? Celebrate. Got our first dollar in revenue? Celebrate. Got our first press coverage? Celebrate. Celebrate might mean pizza and beers in the afternoon. Or it might mean a barbeque cooked to order for the team by the executives, or an outing at a lake for everyone's families. We always took Halloween very seriously and turned the event into a competition. Departments transformed their portions of the offices into thematic storybook lands and judges chose which department had done the most creative job. (I would get competitive here, too, and always tried to win.) We also had the most aggressive, competitive volleyball team. We used lunchtime games not just to celebrate, but also to let off the steam of constant startup pressure-cooking.

After a couple of startups, I expected and assumed all of these behaviors. But when I first went from being a university professor at an institution born in the 1920s to a startup born the week before I arrived, it was all new to me. The biggest shock was finding that everyone else on the team wanted me to succeed, not fail. At a university, either you have tenure or you don't. In most departments, if you don't have tenure, you have to get it within six years or you are required to leave. The number of junior faculty competing for the few choice tenure slots is much greater than the number of slots. This creates an environment of unhealthy competition for those slots: the others rather openly relish each and every setback and failure you have because it increases their odds of making it. In stark and pleasant contrast, at a startup anyone else's failure directly hurts you and your ownership stake in the enterprise. The minute you have a setback at a startup, others jump in to help you fix what is wrong or catch up if you have gotten behind. I suppose this must feel somewhat like a soldier in the battlefield, where every man who goes down hurts the chances of the whole unit.

Startup teams are different from any other type of working group I have ever seen. They are like good sports teams. My best startup teams were like my best whitewater rafting team: a well-oiled machine where each individual knew what everyone else was thinking and what they would do next. I wanted to lead such teams simply because I wanted to accomplish more than I could do on my own. When you go from being an individual contributor implementing your ideas to a leader driving a team to implement those same ideas, you magnify the possibilities dramatically. That is the essence of a startup: to think and act as one, with a common goal, intense focus, and a determination to reach the goal as fast as possible.

I was on the edge all the time. It felt like I had converged my extreme sports persona and my career persona—seamlessly. A startup is fragile. There is a clock on your money ticking relentlessly away, and the money will run out if you don't get enough from customers in time. In that case, you have to go back to the well and get more money from investors. Going back to investors translates into great pain because they take another big chunk of ownership in your company and make demands with which you can't argue. Each time you go to them, you lose more control of your baby, up to the point where you are shoved out the door. However, if the product is not ready or has not had enough time to gain traction in the marketplace, there is no other option.

My emotions were running very high about having to leave WorldCert. These were stronger emotions than I had felt since I was nineteen and learned that the cancer had spread from leg to lung. But I was an optimist. I looked forward and knew the next one would be much better. The next one was called WebServices.

On a therapeutic bike ride north of Boston, I rode by a father and son biking together. Something about the father nagged at me for several hundred yards. Then it hit me that he was a dead ringer for someone I had worked with at Borland ten years before, back in California. It seemed hard to believe that same person could be out biking in a tiny Boston suburb on my bike route, but the recognition was strong enough that I decided to turn around. With a little more gray hair than I remembered, it was indeed Dan O'Connor out with his son. He had become a recruiter and, of course, wanted to know if I was employed. When I told him that I had just become unemployed, he excitedly suggested introducing me to his friend—a VC—Richard.

Richard was a partner at a new VC firm in Boston and was looking at doing a deal that needed a technical CEO to lead it. It was in an area I knew a fair amount about as I was still in the middle of writing a book about that topic. Richard wanted me to quickly meet the technical founders of a group calling themselves "WebServices." On the day of the meeting, I went to Richard's office and was sitting with him in his large conference room when in walked the entire team that had helped me found Webspective in 1997. Richard knew this was my old team but, in the interest of creating a dramatic reunion, he kept it secret. He wanted to see how we all reacted and whether this would be a good match. That, in turn, would help him decide if it was a team he wanted to bet on. I was pretty excited, and it was all happening so fast after my departure from the last startup. Next I had to meet Richard's co-investor, Dick, from the bigger VC firm.

Dick seemed like Mr. Nice Guy, but he had an edge. He was almost so nice it was hard to trust him, but his charm disarmed you from being too suspicious. Upon meeting me, he immediately launched into how I was not the long-term CEO of this new venture. "Oh, but you are the perfect CEO right now," he said. "But when we decide the time is right, we are going to bring someone in to take over the thing you will have built up." I like the early phase best anyway because that is when you are doing pure invention. Still, the specter of some unknown person coming in and taking over our "baby" in eighteen months felt like walking down a dark alley, constantly looking over your shoulder to see who might be following you.

In spite of looking over my shoulder, the early phase, like at the other startups, was fun and creative. There was no market for what we were building, but we were optimistic that there would be and that we could help create it. We searched for customers to validate that we were building something they wanted to buy. We got the first round of money, and as we burned through that money and still had no revenue from customers, we needed to get more money. About fifteen months into the company's life, Dick said it was about time to start the search for a new CEO.

The investors chose a new CEO who had only worked as chief technical officer at big companies, had never run sales or marketing, and had never raised money. All five founders, including me, instead wanted someone who knew sales and marketing. But Dick wanted the big company technical guy. Since he controlled our access to cash, he alone decided who was to be the CEO.

I remained for a year helping the new CEO. After I left, the company ran out of cash and had to shut down. WebServices never got the chance to be successful—a story that is all too common in the world of high tech, venture capital-backed startups.

My optimism and my resilience were being sorely tested. I treated this much the same way I treated the process of learning to ski fast down a steep field of moguls on one ski. Keep at it. Never give up. Again, I gained strength from reminding myself that nothing I would go though in business could compare to the death threat I had received when I was nineteen.

I needed to move on to something new and exciting. Right then, Dave Chen, my co-founder of WorldCert, who was now a venture capitalist himself, called and asked for my help on his newest investment idea. He was considering investing in PetaBric, a startup in Portland, Oregon, which was building a microprocessor designed for ultra-high performance applications, like encoding and decoding the HD television signals sent down the cable to our TV sets. Dave wanted me to evaluate the technology behind the company to help him decide if it was a good investment. I said I just was not sure I was the right guy to evaluate a chip company.

"It's all math and you were a math major," he said.

"Yes, but that was thirty years ago. And it's not all math. They are designing a hardware chip."

"Well, you did your PhD on designing computer chips, didn't you?"

"That was in 1983. I think the technology might have advanced since then," I frustratingly quipped. But I had already resigned to saying yes.

The company had brilliant hardware people—especially the co-founder, who was the hardware CTO, but was very weak on its software. This was a huge problem because a chip needs applications programmed for it, and those programmers need tools, which only the chip company can provide. On my recommendation, Dave did invest in the company, but then asked if I would come out for a week and assess how they should best address their software shortcomings. That sounded like fun, would pay well, and would get me involved with something very technically challenging. While there, the other founder and the new CEO tried hard to persuade me to join the company as their software CTO. They wanted me to get the software side of their business staffed up and organized. It was so interesting and so new and different that I actually agreed to commute 2,700 miles across country for a year. It meant that Carole and I were apart two weeks out of three. I didn't get too lonely during the week because I worked long hours. But the weekends were a drag. It was during that time that I decided to write this book.

While flying across the country every one to two weeks and living alone in a furnished apartment was torture, getting back to being very technical was both refreshing and a confidence builder. It had been a long time since I had rolled up my technical sleeves, but I was able to hold my own and make a real contribution. I better organized the people we had and started aggressively hiring to fill in the most critical open spots. I also dove into the technical work of designing the software we had to build and provide to our customers. This involved the mind-bending work of understanding how to harness the power of some three hundred or so processors on a single chip without totally blowing the mind of a developer trying to use our software to build an application to run on that chip.

As frequently happens on engineering projects, especially new hardware designs, events did not follow the best-laid plans and pre-determined schedule. In fact, things slipped over six months during the one year I was there. This was made worse by continuous design changes in response to improvements the hardware CTO kept making. The project was going out of control. Still, progress was made and the chip was slowly laid out by the physical designers. The physical designers practiced a mysterious black art; they programmed where the silicon should be etched to create the microscopic transistors, several hundred million of which would eventually have to be perfectly constructed to make a working chip. One mistake can destroy a chip worth hundreds of thousands of dollars in fabrication costs and six months of time. Tests, checks, and crosschecks were constantly made, all in software, to verify that the chip, if laid out precisely as specified, would indeed work as designed. In the final step before sending the physical design specification file to the chip foundry in Taiwan, we applied a set of strict design rules (provided from the foundry) to the layout to tie that layout to the physical realities of the particular chip fabrication process. It was absolutely critical that we applied these rules just as the foundry specified them. Otherwise, the foundry would not guarantee that the chips would work and the hundreds of thousands of dollars we paid to them for the run would be wasted.

Something was wrong. The chip did not run fast enough to meet our minimal design requirements. But suddenly and miraculously, over a weekend, things converged and to everyone's relief the simulated chip started to work correctly. On Monday, we encrypted the bits to keep them safe, and then sent them over the Internet to the Taiwan foundry. In just a matter of weeks, we would have chips back and everyone was pretty sure they would work. But to our horror, when the foundry got our bits and did their standard final sanity check, they reported that something was amiss. They figured out that we had changed the specifications of their physical process. The one thing we were not allowed to change. We were supposed to consider their design rules sacrosanct and change our design until it all worked with their rules for their process. Someone had changed their files to define their process differently, and this was what had made our design magically start to work. Mysteriously, the co-founder CTO left the company quietly the next day. In spite of this tragedy, I had built a software team that, in turn, had built a programming environment for this chip that customers loved. And when the chip finally was built and did work, the company got a lot of customers who were very happy with the work we had done.

I told the CEO and the board that I would finish the year I had committed to, but on the anniversary date I would leave. They were not happy and fought to keep me. That was nice to hear, but I couldn't keep doing that commute. That year had seemed like the longest in my career. And all the efforts ended up being for naught. Three years later, when PetaBric needed more money to keep going, a bad economy caused the VCs to withhold further funding. This killed PetaBric fast and hard.

After a steady diet of startups and VCs for thirteen years, I felt like I had learned an important lesson: VCs will be VCs, and expecting them to act differently is unrealistic. It was a hard-fought lesson, just like the timeless lesson of "The Little Boy and the Rattlesnake" parable, as told by Cherokee, Seneca, and Hindo peoples:

> *The little boy was walking down a path and he came across a rattlesnake. The rattlesnake was getting old. He asked, "Please little boy, can you take me to the top of the mountain? I hope to see the sunset one last time before I die." The little boy answered "No, Mr. Rattlesnake. If I pick you up, you'll bite me and I'll die." The rattlesnake said, "No, I promise. I won't bite you. Just please take me up to the mountain." The little boy thought about it and finally picked up that rattlesnake and took it close to his chest and carried it up to the top of the mountain.*
>
> *They sat there and watched the sunset together. It was so beautiful. Then after the sunset, the rattlesnake turned to the little boy and asked, "Can I go home now? I am tired, and I am old." The little boy picked up the rattlesnake and again took it to his chest and held it tightly and safely. He came all the way down the mountain, holding the snake carefully, and took it to his home to give him some food and a place to sleep. The next day the rattlesnake turned to the boy and asked, "Please little boy, will you take me back to my home now? It is time for me to leave this world, and I would like to be at my home now." The little boy felt he had been safe all this time and the snake had kept his word, so he would take him home as asked.*

He carefully picked up the snake, took it close to his chest, and carried him back to the woods, to his home, to die. Just before he laid the rattlesnake down, the rattlesnake turned and bit him in the chest. The little boy cried out and threw the snake upon the ground. "Mr. Snake, why did you do that? Now I will surely die!" The rattlesnake looked up at him and grinned, "You knew what I was when you picked me up."

Like the little boy with the snake, I consistently forgot what the VCs really were. But unlike the boy, when I was "bitten," I survived to fight again. Now it seems that I've stopped fighting that fight and accepted things as they are, just as I've stopped taking on every single challenge and dare thrown down at me as a way of fighting back from the disability. It took decades to stop looking over my shoulder, to stop taking on every physical and career challenge, to relax and just live like there really was a tomorrow. Maybe I'm not so incorrigible after all.

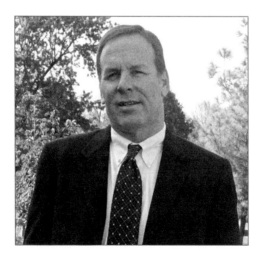

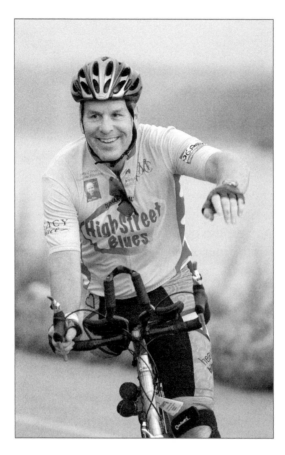

ACCIDENTAL INSPIRATION

Hope, as opposed to cynicism and despair, is the sole precondition for a new and better life.

— William Sloane Coffin, clergyman/activist

We make a living by what we get; we make a life by what we give.

— Sir Winston Churchill, politician

Initially, sports were the key to regaining my self-esteem. Downhill skiing, waterskiing, rafting, crutch hiking, open water swimming. They gave me satisfaction; they fed my love of speed and excitement; and most importantly they allowed me to attain the status of "not considering."

Notwithstanding the little bit of biking around our circle road in North Carolina and the occasional tandem ride with Carole along the ocean in California, biking was not a major factor in my life until we settled in Boston.

Most people can't envision how one-legged biking works. Getting on a bike is easy. Without an extra leg to lift all the way over the seat and cross bar, I can just edge onto the seat from the side on which I am standing. The bike does not have to be perfectly vertical to balance. (Think about what they do with trick bikes in the circus.) When going very slowly, the bike can lean a little to one side, as long as the upper body is compensating by leaning out over the bike to the side opposite the way the bike is tipped. I have learned to balance in this way naturally and instinctively. After mounting the bike, I just push off with the foot on the ground to get moving, and then I clip the foot cleat that is on the bottom of my bike shoe into the pedal and start pulling up and pushing down. As the bike gains speed, the large wheels act like gyroscopes. If you took one of those gyroscope toys we had as kids, got it spinning fast, and held just the tip in your hand with the wheel spinning vertically, you would not easily be able to bump that wheel away from vertical. A bike's wheels are very large, relative to the size and weight of the bike. When they are spinning fast, the gyroscope effect is very stabilizing, even with an extra twenty to twenty-five pounds on one side. When I slow way down getting ready to stop, I have to be careful not to lean to the side where there is no leg. Once the bike starts to tip that way, I am pretty helpless to do anything because there is no leg on that side to catch me. I just wait for the ground to rise up and hit me. Hard. I only made that mistake a couple of times. Instead, as the bike loses its momentum and the gyroscope effect dies down, I lean slightly toward my legged side as I unclip my foot from the pedal. I reach my toe down to the ground just as the bike comes to a stop. Of course, it's even better if I can find a stop sign or parking signpost to grab onto. It is much easier to start from a dead stop, clipped into the pedal, than it is to push on the ground fast enough to coast a ways while I find the clip. This is also why it is near impossible to start going up a hill. If I find myself stopping facing uphill, I typically have to turn around, ride a few yards downhill until I am well clipped in, and then do a quick U-turn back to where I started. Learning all this did take time and practice, though now it is second nature.

Toe clips or cleats allow me a strong pull up as well as a push down on each stroke, and I develop the pull-up part of the stroke to a much greater extent than two-leggers. The tough question is how do I build up strength in a single leg to be able to ride one hundred miles in a single day? I do not know enough about exercise physiology to understand this, so it remains a mystery to me. I know that, like swimming, I have to work harder at the beginning of every season than any two-legged rider. If I lay off riding (or any of my activities), even for a little while, I have to fight hard to get the strength back. While I am working out to get strong for the endurance events, I focus very hard and tend to work best by myself. It's something hard and lonely I just need to get through.

The little biking I had done before, I liked a lot. It felt good to build my leg muscles, it gave me an addictive endorphin rush, and I liked the speed and freedom it offered. But I never pushed beyond a few laps on our little circle road in North Carolina.

Once we were in Boston and the kids were no longer interested in biking with us, we never rode much and any conscious thought about biking slowly waned. But after about three years, I began hearing about the AIDS research rides, which were long rides to raise money and awareness for AIDS. Ironically, it took my moving to the opposite coast for me to learn about fundraising rides that actually originated in California. Their seminal event was a seven-day ride from San Francisco to Los Angeles. Carole had worked extensively with AIDS patients in Santa Cruz, where many were dying on a weekly basis. Now in Boston, she was again dealing with AIDS in the homeless population. Fortunately, dramatic progress had been made and people with HIV were living much longer because of new, potent antiretroviral drugs. Like chemotherapy, those life-preserving drugs came out of research. Research takes a lot of money, so I always felt generous when it came to giving money to AIDS-related causes.

Sarah, who worked for Novasoft when I was the CEO, asked if I would sponsor her in the local edition AIDS ride. She was going to ride her bike from Boston to New York City. It would take four days to go the 375 miles, and she needed to raise a minimum of $1,500 to participate. Not only was I impressed with the feat itself, but also with the organization that was creating so many rides in cities across the country and was raising money for a cause I considered so vital. I enthusiastically sponsored her.

I kept asking Sarah how she would train, what she expected the ride to be like, and how hard she thought it would be. Sarah was an athlete, for sure. I knew she ran, rollerbladed, and rode, but she did not seem like a fanatic. This was 375 miles. I was totally impressed. Certainly driving a car four and a half hours to New York didn't equate in my mind to something normal people could do on a bike.

After Sarah did the ride, I wanted to know everything. That year, however, Boston had a direct hit from the remnants of a gulf coast hurricane during her ride. So all I heard was that the ride was terrible due to the rain and wind and having to be bussed over major portions of the route because the hurricane was wreaking havoc on all the riders.

Still, I could not stop talking about it. I was proud to have been a sponsor and have my money go to AIDS research. Then I heard the assertion that changed my life. I don't even recall who said it. "That is impressive," this person said, "but I bet someone with one leg could never do that." As I had many times before, I thought, *Who says I can't?*

That simple statement became my battle cry. I told Carole the AIDS ride was my new goal. I asked to have the bike back I had given to her in North Carolina. I can't say whether she thought I was crazy, or could never pull this off, or what. Outwardly, Carole was her normal, supportive self. The ride was in late summer, so I started training as early in the spring as one can in New England.

First, I did a little four-mile ride from the house. That turned out to be quite easy, which was a pleasant surprise. I wondered why I had waited so long to try riding in a more serious way. I found a nice loop of eleven miles around Boston College. That was a little harder and tired my leg, especially the muscles that pull up on the pedal.

I now had a vision that I could build up to greater and greater distances. I was still scared of what I had committed to because eleven miles or twenty-five miles is nothing like 375 miles. And I had no idea about hills yet. I did some local hills, but I knew these were piddling compared to what I would face in Connecticut. Even so, I hit a couple of hills on training rides that I just did not have enough gas to climb. On really tough hills, or when they are very tired, two-leggers stand up on their pedals or—as a final resort— get off the bike and walk it up the rest of the hill. With one leg, I cannot stand up on the pedals; I must do every hill sitting in the saddle. And since I can't get off and walk (or hop) up such a hill, there is no option but to turn around to go back down to the flats to rest. There I would have to rest long enough to be able to make it all the way up the hill on my second try. I did not want any "do overs" during the AIDS ride, partly because it would add to my distance, but mostly because it would be humiliating.

I slowly worked my way up to twenty-five-, then thirty-five-, then forty-five-mile training rides. My leg was getting a real workout and gaining more endurance. By the end of each of these training rides, I struggled the last few miles. The energy seemed to ooze out of me, my speed dropped, and it became harder and harder to make it up even gradual inclines. My bike computer displayed my current speed, my average speed, and my total distance ridden. As exhaustion set in, insidiously my speed began to drop. It felt like I was still working just as hard, but there was not as much power coming from each push-pull. I took advantage of every opportunity to coast so my muscles could recover. I was very uncomfortable.

In pain, you might say. In many sports, one of the huge benefits of two legs is that one gets a tiny bit of rest while the other one does most of the work, and then they switch roles. That is certainly true in cycling. Even good cyclists ease off the pull-up when their legs become fatigued. Frequently at high levels of exhaustion, there is a mental effect as well. I can best describe it as a minor disorientation. It is subtle and seeps in slowly. Unless I bonk.

Bonking is when the body literally runs out of fuel. I had never before done any kind of physical activity that ran the risk of bonking, but it is common in long distance cycling and marathon running. In an instant, my energy would drop to nearly zero. From a steady fourteen or fifteen miles per hour, I suddenly struggled to maintain even nine or ten miles per hour. Unless you have experienced bonking and know what to expect, it is hard to recognize it happening, partly because the disorientation affects the brain as well as the body. You need food.

Biking made me realize how much my body is like a machine. I needed to provide it with food and water to survive long bike rides. I found that training rides of fifty miles or less were survivable with just a couple of water bottles full of water and a granola bar midway along. Longer than that and I needed to carry some real food, like peanut butter sandwiches and fruit, as well as a backpack of water. With a training ride of more than fifty miles, I worked many of my body's muscles very hard for four or more hours.

After doing long rides for seven years, when I had always lived by the rule I had to ride to the top of any hill I started up no matter what, I found the exception to the rule while working in Portland, Oregon. At the corporate apartment where I lived when I was there, I kept a bike for training rides. I had mapped out a route for a weekend ride that I thought would be fun. It went up to the road that runs along the spine of the boundary ridge outside Portland called Skyline Drive. I was going to gut it out climbing up that hill, ride along Skyline enjoying its spectacular views, and then ride back down where I would get a thrilling (and restful) fast coasting ride back down to the valley floor. As I started to climb, my speed dropped, I put the bike into the lowest of the low gears and concentrated on a steady pace of pull up, push down. The terrain ahead changed; I could see that I was going to have a downhill run for a bit before the real climb to the top began. Just as I started to coast down the hill, the pavement ended. I had to slow down quickly to avoid a nasty skid on the gravel. Riding my brakes the rest of the way down, I kept my speed down and hoped that the pavement restarted soon. At the bottom of this little valley there was a paved bridge over a creek that fooled me into a false sense of relief. No such luck. The pavement was just for the span length of the bridge. Not only did the pavement end again, but as the temporary sign pointed out, the gravel was fresh and loose too. A few hard pumps of my pedal confirmed just how loose that gravel was. My back wheel just spun in place. I stopped moving completely, in spite of pedaling hard. I had to react quickly. I clipped out of my pedal to avoid a painful fall to one side and then stood up next to my bike. I looked up the gravel hill in front of me. As far as I could see was soft, fresh gravel. I looked back up the hill that I had just descended. More soft, fresh gravel. I was screwed. I could not ride up the hill behind me or the one in front of me. I tried to pedal again several times to see if there was a softer technique that would allow me to get traction and make forward progress.

No cars were anywhere to be seen, and I am not sure I would have asked them for help if there had been. I had a cell phone, but that was just for real emergencies. Calling someone to get me out of this situation would feel just too embarrassing. I had only one option. I was going to have to do what I said must never happen: hop up that hill. There was no sense in hopping back the way I had come, since that would not get me in the right direction. But I had no idea how far I would have to hop in the direction I was heading. After all, the mapping program had not told me this was an unpaved road in the first place. I found I could hop about fifty hops before I needed to rest for a few minutes. That, according to my bike computer, was eleven hundredths of a mile or about thirty-five yards. It was very slow going and extremely frustrating. When faced with a situation with only one solution, I always find it best to just suck it up and get through it. In the end, I hopped almost two miles. The road twisted and turned and got steeper and flatter, so I could never see how much further I had to hop. Sometimes I tried to lean harder on the bike to give my leg a break. Sometimes I thought the gravel seemed more packed or the pitch was not very great, and

I tried getting back on the bike to ride again. No luck. There was just no other option but to hop fifty hops, rest, and repeat. Finally, after hopping for close to an hour, I saw the pavement I had been hoping for around every bend in the road. Once back on the bike, I still had a lot of climbing to do and then a long way beyond that to get back to the apartment. My leg was shot compared to how it felt before the hopping. Unfortunately, my apartment was on the third floor of a building with no elevator. I had acknowledged that I had to hop up and down those two flights of stairs with my bike whenever I went for a ride, but this time it was much, much harder to get my leg to do those last few dozen stair hops with the bike. For several days, my calf muscle reminded me of my misjudgment on that particular training ride.

Not far from my house back in Boston, where I knew which roads were paved, was one of the steepest hills I had ever seen. It was not long, but it was extremely steep. I felt it would boost my confidence and build up my leg's hill climbing ability if I did some work on that hill. So I set a schedule and a goal, as I do for almost everything I tackle. Once a week, I would include this hill at the end of one of my shorter training routes. And not just one trip up this hill, mind you. Each week, I would add one iteration of the hill to my routine. According to my plan, I would pedal up that hill ten times in a row the week before the big event.

The hill was right in front of the kid's high school. I shifted my bike into its lowest "granny" gear and started my ascent. By the halfway point, I was panting hard and still had a ways to go. My speed dropped precipitously to the point—as low as four miles per hour—where I was barely able to keep the bike upright. I always did this ride in the early morning when there was little traffic. When I got to the very top, I took a big swig of water, gave myself a bit of a ride on the flat to recover, and then turned around to fly down the hill. This hill was so steep I couldn't just let the bike go or I'd be going fifty miles per hour by the time I reached the bottom and would be unable to stop. I rode the brakes all the way down to the bottom. Then I shifted all the way down to low gear and did it again. The few people out running or walking their dogs no doubt wondered what I was doing.

I worked up to seventy-mile rides before that first AIDS ride. On a ride that long, my average speed is usually about fourteen miles per hour. That is five hours in the saddle—five solid hours of one leg alternately pounding down and pulling up. Around Boston, it is hard to find a really good cycling route that long. The best ones— where it is easy to keep off main roads and increase my chances of surviving the occasional maniacal motorists in Boston—are no more than forty-five miles. The longer routes put me on major roads like Route 20 or Route 117 that head west out of the Boston suburbs near our home.

That summer of training for my first AIDS ride, I was still riding the old steel-frame bike that had been mine, then Carole's, and then mine again. It was now twelve years old. We were riding on Mt. Desert Island with Eric and Cristin during one of our former PA group vacations when Eric said he could see the whole frame of the bike flex on each powerful down stroke I made when climb- ing a hill. He was certain the frame was going to break soon at high speed, which could be disastrous. That prompted Carole to do something totally out of character as a frugal Midwestern girl. She insisted on having a custom bike made for me at a cost of more than $5,000. Other than a car, she had never spent that much on any one item before. She was convinced I was fully committed to this bike-riding thing and that it would be a good investment. We had each experienced desire for items that we thought we wanted, but after we purchased it our interest waned and the money was wasted. My biking to fundraise seemed different to her. She felt it was tightly linked to my leg, my lung, my survival, and my growing desire to give back. And that, she figured, was not a passing fad. She was right.

The frame of my new custom bike was made of titanium. When they welded it together to match the exact dimensions from the mockup on which they measured me, they double-welded strate- gic joints to make sure my one-sided pounding would not stress or unduly flex it. A perfectly-fitting bike changed my rides dramati- cally. I could ride faster, farther, longer. They installed a special set of gears so that I had very low gears for the steeper hills. They put a tandem wheel on the back because, since I did not ever stand up to pedal, my constant weight on the seat stressed the rear wheel to the point where spokes broke. My new bike felt absolutely perfect to me. My average speed jumped by two miles per hour, due to the fit and smooth riding. I could even attach my crutches, which collapsed into three parts that fit on a rack over my rear wheel.

Jerry Walters, who worked with me at WorldCert, was a fanatic cyclist. His hero in life was Eddie Meryx, who had won more Tour de France's than anyone else until Lance Armstrong came along and did it seven times. Jerry was going to join me on the AIDS ride. I was quite relieved to have a companion to share the ride and who would be able to carry things like tents and gear when we stopped for the night to camp. My collapsible crutches were forearm crutches, not full-arm-length crutches, which meant I could not free up a hand to carry something like a plate of food by squeezing the arm pad with my armpit. On our first training ride together, I was amazed to find that Jerry and I were very compatible riders. We rode at exactly the same speed. I expected any rider with whom I rode to pull away from me on each hill because of how much my speed declined. However, this was not an issue with Jerry, and we stayed glued to each other's wheels even on twenty- or thirty-mile rides.

The AIDS ride began in downtown Boston before dawn. Carole took Jerry and me to the starting spot. I was very nervous. I kept thinking about what might happen on the first major hill. *What if I could not make it up and had to stop? Would I make it all the way to the first night's campsite, or would I have to be brought in via the sag wagon? What about day two? Once my leg got good and tired, would I have enough to do it all over again?*

While we waited around for the event to start, I stretched to keep myself busy and loose. When I'm nervous, I become very focused and quiet, so I didn't pay much attention to the stares. They were usually the typical glance, followed by the classic double take. Some people just stared when they were pretty sure I wouldn't notice.

Speeches made, tires pumped, muscles loose, bladders emptied for the umpteenth time. The time arrived for 2,500 riders to depart the campus of Northeastern University in Boston and head for New York City. Carole joined the throngs lined up along our exit route. The start was slow and methodical, with riders funneling through a narrow opening onto the street. Even though it was dawn, cops were out in force at every intersection to help the throngs of riders breeze through red lights. Just as we got out onto the streets of Boston, it started to drizzle. All I had was a light windbreaker, so if it rained hard, I was going to get soaked. I was not too concerned.

It was September, so I knew it wouldn't get too cold, and I would generate enough heat by riding hard. With stories of heavy rain on previous AIDS rides, I should have been more concerned.

We slowly made our way out Beacon Street past Boston College, through Newton, and within a few blocks of my home. From there, we went through Wellesley and Dover as we began to veer south. The rain started to come down very hard. Glasses were of no use. They would get an almost opaque water film on them, yet without glasses the driving rain stung my eyes. The rest stops were quickly becoming lakes, but they were still a respite from the driving rain. All the riders, no matter what they wore, were soaked to the bone. Everyone needed to stop, but we knew if we stopped too long our bodies would chill and we would just delay the long ride ahead of us. The first night's camp was all the way deep into Connecticut, on the campus of the University of Connecticut in the middle of a set of fierce hills.

The first hill test was shortly after we crossed the border into Connecticut on a little road that roughly parallels I-84. By then, the 2,500 riders stretched out over miles as the difference between the fast riders, who insisted this was a race, and the slowest riders, who knew it wasn't, continued to magnify. Many of the slowest riders had not trained. They rode on what looked like borrowed bikes, in many cases mountain bikes or beat up old three speeds. These riders were not athletes, but were driven by the cause. They knew someone who had AIDS and many carried signs and pictures of loved ones lost. I could see it in their eyes. They seemed to feel no pain as they rode mile after mile; some rode continuously for twelve hours to make the ninety miles for that day. They just rode and rode, trying to get somewhere that might somehow help solve this problem that was causing so much pain.

The huge string of riders bunched up at the base of large hills as riders slowed their speed dramatically as they started up the slope. Since these were not interstate highways, the hills were not beaten into submission to become slight up and down grades. The grade on some of these hills was steep, and many were also long. As I approached that first hill and the bunching riders, anxiety got my heart rate going even more than the physical exertion. I had misjudged how fast I would be on these hills. I started to pass riders. Some people got off their bikes and walked up the steeper hills. As I rode past them, Jerry said the stares and double takes were commonplace. I didn't mind. They were for the right reason.

People started to make comments, too.

"You inspire me."

"If you can do it, I have to stop this whining."

"Way to go."

"Tough man."

"Superman!"

I must have passed several hundred people on those hills by the end of the first day. The rest stops were every twenty miles or so, and it was important to fuel up at each one because we were burning a mighty number of calories. Peanut butter sandwiches provided the best fuel. I think we all looked like starving refugees the way we stuffed our mouths with the food laid out on huge platters on the food tables. Even here, random people came up to me to comment. Jerry looked at me afterward and said, "Well, what am I? Chopped liver?" He may as well have been invisible when people approached to encourage or thank me.

From our handlebar-mounted bike computers and the provided route maps, we knew we were close to our goal for the day. But it is very hilly in Storrs, Connecticut, and these organizers had a sadistic streak to test our commitment to the AIDS cause many times a day in the form of extra hills when we were most tired. Home for the night was at the top of a series of very steep hills after we had already gone more than eighty miles. But we made it. I made it. And there were only a few hundred bikes parked ahead of us. We were early. Just as we arrived to settle in our tents to rest and refuel, the rain stopped and the clouds cleared.

They created a veritable tent city for us. One huge tent was for the food. That tent offered multiple stations at which to fill my plate and get drinks. Drinks especially. There were tents for massages, for first aid treatment, for information. There were trucks with our tents and gear in them. There were trucks with kitchens in them. And, most importantly, there were trucks with hot showers in them. These trucks were specially outfitted for smoke jumpers from the west who used them to follow wildfires and to provide respite from their hot, dusty work. They provided us much needed respite from our hard work, too.

I got my collapsible crutches off the back of my bike and happily left my bike in the parking field, not to be touched or thought of until the next day. We found our designated gear truck, got our tent and luggage, set up the tent, and found our shower gear. Once showered and in dry clothes sipping a cold drink, I reflected on what I had just accomplished. I had gone from being knocked flat by the loss of a leg and a lung and all that went with that, to this. To now. To a place where I was motivating people to work harder and become more determined. They told me I was an inspiration to them. *An inspiration?* I had never conceived of being any such thing. In fact, I would never in a million years have thought of applying that word to myself.

A woman came up to me and told me, "You put me in the hospital." But she said it with a smile, so I waited for the punch line. She continued, "You passed me on a hill. That fired me up and I gave it all I had to follow you up that hill. But when I got to the top, I collapsed in exhaustion. The sag wagon had to take me to the hospital. But I am happy because you made me push myself harder than I thought possible." Then she gave me a big hug.

Dozens of people saw me crutch walking around camp and made comments. On the ride and here in camp, the energy from the other riders was affecting me in a way I had never anticipated. I was in awe of the friendliness of this group of strangers. They all had a purpose. They were willing to pay a price in sweat and pain to feel good about that purpose. And they had profound respect for my contribution to that purpose. Because they were riders, they knew how hard I had worked to get ready for this. They knew I was going through more pain than they were. Perhaps in the course of a workout, they had tried one-legged riding. Even serious riders who try one-legged riding don't sustain it for very long and would never try a hill that way. So they respected what I had just accomplished. The fact that I was inspiring these people was a totally new concept to me and it was just beginning to register. I still did not know quite what to make of it. It was not something I had anticipated or sought. The truth is, while the AIDS cause was a huge motivator, I was really doing this for me. When I thought about my personal motivations, I felt guilty. But the reactions from all these people made me realize I could realign my purpose.

It was not just the people in the ride. The towns along the way got out in force to cheer us on. Those people, too, were affected by AIDS, and this cause was important enough to get them out to cheer on some tired, wobbly riders. One of the sights that brought cheers and tears was the group of "positive peddlers." A large group of HIV-positive riders stayed together as a group called a peloton. Those people were sick. Some had seriously diminished lung function. Some had other, more serious, symptoms of AIDS. But they rode. And many of them rode very hard. When some of them came up to give me hugs for helping their cause, I told them that what they were doing was way more impressive than what I was doing. They would have none of that. Regardless, I was inspired by their willingness to fight through being sick, feeling short of breath, being weak from the illness and the medicines, all because they were so committed to the cause. They were going to do this no matter what until they were on their death bed.

Day two was difficult. Everyone's legs really wanted a rest day, yet off we went at the crack of dawn for another ninety miles to another town in Connecticut. By the third day, our bodies adapted to the new level of work, and it almost seemed to get easier. Besides, the names of the towns told us we were getting ever closer to the Big Apple, so the psychological lift helped too.

When we crossed into Manhattan on day four, there was a huge change in our environment. Instead of small towns with people lining the street, cheering us on, passing us water, and even throwing us M&Ms, we now had taxis and buses trying to cut us off. New York streets are for them, not for bikes, they were telling us in a not-so-subtle way. We all had our scary moments on these NYC streets. I even heard taxi drivers shout out of their windows, "Get the fuck off my road."

Our destination was an auditorium on Eighth Avenue. Here we could all collect, rest, and refuel while waiting for every last rider to join us so we could all ride the final stretch together. Jerry and I were near the front of the group riding into Manhattan because, by the fourth day, my leg had gotten even stronger, and I could push as hard as all but the elite racers.

Once everyone arrived, we all got back on our bikes for our final processional. Eighth Avenue was closed just for us. The sides were packed with well-wishers. It was a ticker tape parade. We slowly proceeded five blocks down Eighth toward a huge stage set up in the middle of the street. Once assembled, the final speeches were given. Speakers shared their sentiments about the scourge of AIDS and how important our task was and how great our accomplishment. These comments had a special double meaning for me. Tears welled up in my eyes. I was deeply moved and I was extremely proud. Carole was there to cheer me on and take me home. In a powered vehicle, thank God!

I was hooked. The whole experience was like a drug. I had not set out to inspire people. I had set out to prove something to myself. To rise to the challenge. To test myself. To renew my frequently-challenged confidence. To feel good about myself. But along the way, people let me know how strongly they felt about what I had accomplished. That recognition and the concept of inspiring others was humbling. Being humbled is not something most people that knew me thought possible. I immediately made plans to do the ride again the next year. They announced the ride would reverse direction from now on, starting near New York and ending in Boston; riding with Manhattan taxis really had been too dangerous to try again.

The next year the ride started in Newburgh, New York. The hills there are much bigger than in Connecticut, and we still had all of Connecticut to pass through, as well. I knew how to prepare for this ride, and I had the confidence of experience behind me. However, it did not lessen the impact of how people on the ride reacted to me.

A large portion of riders on the AIDS rides was gay. Once the morning horde spreads out to a long single file, a natural selection quickly sorts the riders according to their speed. Riders then tend to ride with the same people throughout the day. Jerry and I met Brian, Andy, and Joanne this way. We kept seeing them at rest stops and on the road. Sometimes we would pass them, but they would be right on our tails, and we'd see them again at the next rest stop. Inevitably, we joined their group. They had lots of questions about my situation, and I was just as curious about how they dealt with the challenges in their lives.

All of them were happy to talk about when they discovered they were gay, when they told their parents, and what their parents' reactions were. Brian summed up the group's sentiments best when he said, "You know, being gay cannot be a choice because no one in their right mind would choose this pain." Andy was the aggressive rider in the group, and I liked riding with him because he pushed me hard. Andy taught me what kind of man he found attractive, so when we passed helpful cops at intersections directing us safely through, I would help Andy spot the ones that matched his taste. I found myself yelling to Andy, "Look at that hottie," in reference to a very manly officer in uniform. Brian, a bigwig at a financial services company, had been a Marine, but since then had come out. Andy was a high school teacher and had not come out. Together, Brian and Andy had adopted two boys. Joanne was a school principal. Also with this group was Dave, with whom I worked. Dave had a below-knee amputation. The one-leggedness was a complete coincidence, but his being on the ride was not. Dave had been an out of shape smoker and had been inspired by what I was doing, so he decided to try it himself. He rode with his prosthesis because his knee gave him a lot of power, plus the leg helped him at rest stops and in camp.

The whole group stayed together for the entire trip. It made this edition of the AIDS ride an even better experience for me. When we got close to Boston, we were on my training routes. I picked up the pace. At twenty miles per hour, all of us in a line, we came screaming into Boston. At the finish at City Hall Square, we all stood in a group, and everyone held up one leg and tucked it behind them for a picture. We called our group "The One-Leggers" from then on. We did one more AIDS ride from New York to Boston the following year. But it was our last AIDS ride. The overall charitable giving of the event dropped below fifty percent. Donors who discovered that quickly dropped out. Donors did not want half the money they donated to be used for overhead. I needed to find a better ride. Fundraising was now a part of my life, as well as Carole's. Plus, I was killing three birds with one stone. One, the athletic events gave me a focus and a goal for keeping in tiptop shape. Two, the events helped inspire people, which I found both motivational and addictive. And, three, the donors I appealed to were generous because they felt good about donating to a great cause and they enjoyed participating vicariously

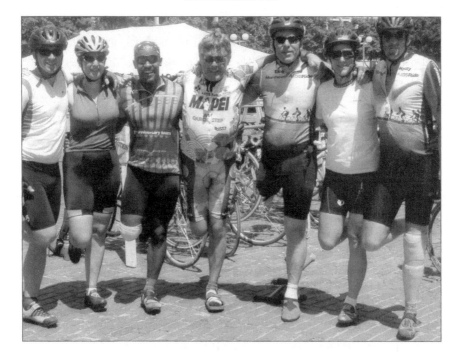

through me. This became even more the case when I switched to two cancer-related bike-riding fundraisers.

Right after the Sydney Olympics, which was right after his fifth Tour de France win, Lance Armstrong was the featured speaker at a software company's conference where I was a technical presenter. The software company's CEO, whom I had befriended, was a triathlon fanatic who knew Lance. He made sure the two of us met. I got only a few moments with Lance, but I outlined my story. He was especially impressed with my being a thirty-year survivor of metastasized cancer. At the time, he was a five-year survivor. I give Lance enormous credit for making it acceptable to use the word *metastases*. When I was a kid, people didn't even talk about cancer, much less admit that cancer had spread within their body. That gradually changed as people realized they couldn't catch cancer from others and that more and more people were surviving cancer. Cancer stopped being such a social stigma. But until Lance made it common conversation, the word *metastatic* was still not used. It was like saying you had a death sentence, and that was too socially uncomfortable for people.

Like me, Lance is a survivor of metastatic cancer. In his case, testicular cancer had metastasized to the brain. Long-term survivorship is the whole focus of his Livestrong Foundation. He asked me to commit to coming to Austin for his annual Ride for the Roses, a one-hundred-mile cancer fundraising ride. I said I would. Carole and I did his ride the next three years. It was quite a production for us. We had to rent bike shipping boxes, dismantle and pack two bikes, fly down with them on the plane on a Friday afternoon, and reassemble and test ride our bikes before joining Lance's seven thousand riders for the one-day event. It followed a one-hundred-mile course through the hills around Austin and ended with a very fun party. We saw only a flash of Lance at the start as he blasted off at high speed with his U.S. Postal teammates. The ride was in the spring, and being from Boston, it was difficult to get enough training in beforehand. I always rode unprepared and in great pain, barely eking out the full one hundred miles with my leg exhausted and numb. No sooner did we finish than we had to dismantle and pack up two bikes for the return trip home the next day.

The challenge from my co-worker got me started on the AIDS rides. The challenge from Lance got me focused on cancer fundraising. I put the two together and became part of the oldest, largest, and most efficient athletic fundraiser in the country, the Pan-Massachusetts Challenge bike-a-thon.

I had heard about the Pan-Massachusetts Challenge bike ride. The PMC, as it is called, had become a local institution. It seemed every bike rider I talked to did it. For twenty-five years, it had been growing and now had the Red Sox, Overstock.com, Harpoon Brewery, and many other big sponsors. When I found out that its sole recipient was the Dana-Farber Cancer Institute, I decided to do it. It is a two-day ride of 192 miles. It starts in Sturbridge, which is in the middle of the state. Therefore, it's not exactly pan-Massachusetts, as the people in western Massachusetts will tell you as they roll their eyes. Starting in Sturbridge makes the ride doable in two days, which avoids the expense of multi-night base camps. The Mass Maritime Academy campus on the banks of the Cape Cod Canal is the event's fixed base camp. Almost five thousand riders sign up for this ride. Some leave from Sturbridge, where the first half-day is a series of significant hills; others leave from Wellesley for a flatter course. All converge during the day and end up together, rolling into Bourne for the night at base camp. The PMC sets a high minimum fundraise amount of more than $4,000. But they can get it, and it is why they can raise a total of $35 million with five thousand riders.

My first year, Carole drove me to Sturbridge at 4:30 a.m. on the first day. It is a one-hour drive from our house. A torrential downpour started as we were driving to the event. Of course, the bike was now soaked, and this was looking to be a very wet ride. The sky started lightening just before 6 a.m., and as the crowd was forming for our departure, the rain stopped. It was still a wet surface, but thankfully there was no more rain for the rest of the day.

I knew no one and had no riding partner, but because of the AIDS rides, I knew what to expect. I had trained well and was ready. Along the way, I discovered people I knew but I kept riding by myself, satisfied with just seeing them at the water stops every twenty miles or so.

The PMC is incredibly organized with respect to the routes, cops at intersections, water stops, sag wagons, and everything else the riders need. With one hundred percent of every donated dollar going to the cancer institute, my donors were quite happy and generous again. The PMC is a lot more fun for me than the AIDS rides. To begin with, it goes through towns no more than two hours from my home. More people—seemingly everyone alive—has been touched by cancer, so the crowds are even larger and more appreciative. And while I care deeply about the victims of AIDS and the AIDS cause, with the PMC I am sort of the "poster child" for what the ride is all about. The PMC and its support for The Dana-Farber Cancer Institute are legendary throughout New England. It's been going through the same little towns up to and out on the Cape for thirty years. The townspeople are used to it, and they seem to genuinely love it. Bagpipers help us up Purgatory Hill. A little nowhere road called Cherry Street paints the pavement, has rock bands, banners, and huge, cheering crowds. A summer camp on the Cape plans for weeks to have its kids cheer us on with floats and signs as we fly by on our bikes.

As we rode, people constantly yelled to us, "Thanks for riding." They helped us up hills saying, "This is the top of the last one," even if it was a lie. PMC riders are a more aggressive and serious group of riders than the AIDS riders. This makes them even more appreciative of my feat, as most of them have tried one-legged cycling.

The first day started out hilly and ended long and hard. The Wellesley starters joined the main flow just before the lunch stop. By the time we arrived at the Mass Maritime Academy for our final resting spot of the day, we had gone 110 miles. More than a century ride. My butt was numb. So was my nether region. My leg was beyond exhaustion. Everything hurt. It was purely a matter of gutting it out the last twenty miles or so to get to the finish line. Once there, a huge field served as bike parking. Eventually five thousand bikes would hang by their seats on horizontal metal pipes, filling an entire football field. Near the bikes were the tents, one option for spending the night. Another alternative was the huge ship called the Enterprise, on which the Massachusetts Maritime students learn. It was air-conditioned, but cramped. The last choice—my pick—were the dorms. They packed four same-sex people in a two-person dorm room. The desks served as the additional two beds with thin mattresses thrown on top. We each brought our own pad, sleeping bag, and pillow.

After hitting the showers, it was time for food and drink. The AIDS ride allowed no alcohol, but the PMC had Harpoon Brewery as a sponsor, so a Harpoon tent with all the free beer you wanted was the first place to stop. A huge massage tent with more than sixty tables staffed by volunteer massage therapists was the second stop. They did just fifteen-minute massages. Some people tried to get what is normally a sixty-minute full body massage jammed into fifteen minutes. Bad idea. Here's where I got yet another one-legged advantage: I asked the therapist to focus on my one leg from ankle to hip for the entire time. Fifteen minutes focused solely on the most tired leg of all the 9,999 legs doing the ride truly gave my poor leg a much-deserved treat.

The food was good and plentiful. The air was cool and comfortable, as we were right on the water at the base of Buzzard's Bay. One of the biggest challenges was staying awake long enough so that I wouldn't wake up in the middle of the night. I decided on an 8 p.m. bedtime. Because I was sharing a dorm with three other guys, I wisely remembered anti-snoring earplugs, but it was still hard to sleep on a hard desk. Reveille was at 4:15 so we could get an early start on day two.

After a quick breakfast and a long stretch to get the previous day's kinks out of my poor leg, I hit the road with the earliest group at 5:15. It was still dark. We climbed the huge, man-made hill that was the Bourne Bridge onto the Cape. It was a Sunday morning, so they took over the right lane to make it easy for us to navigate the bridge. On the other side, we looped around underneath the bridge to the bike path along the canal. It went five miles north to the inside of the Cape, where we started to head east out to the Cape proper. We headed right into the sunrise. The bike path is flat and fast. Adrenalin was flowing freely. We were all excited and delighted to be on the Cape. We had eighty miles to go, but it seemed like the end was in reach.

I was passed a lot during the PMC because the riders were so much more competitive than on AIDS rides. Huge groups of riders form long pelotons. They travel as an integrated unit, drafting off each other. Solely focused on their own formation, they were very aggressive and sometimes not particularly friendly. In fact, they were downright dangerous and should have probably been broken up. While peloton after peloton passed me in the gray dawn, I still maintained a speed of more than twenty miles per hour. When the sun infused me with even more energy, I tried to hold back or I risked totally running out of steam hours later.

The Cape is not flat. The roads on the Cape all undulate over ancient sand dunes. Little hills are in many ways harder than long hills. They still kill my speed. I can't stand up to keep my momentum, but when I get to the top, the down slope is equally short and provides little recovery and rest. Even though it was 5:30 on a Sunday morning, the dedicated Cape residents were out in force to cheer us on to the next town. Town after town, we made steady progress on our way to Provincetown.

The Cape first heads east, but then bends north, and finally west, as it loops back on itself. Our route was back roads most of the way until it narrowed to its narrowest point, where only one road existed for all traffic. Once we were out of Wellfleet and past our last water stop, we went over the next rise to Truro. At this point, we could see Provincetown. It looked only a few minutes away. The huge monument to the Pilgrims beckoned to us. But the organizers of the PMC had a final surprise. Just like the AIDS ride organizers, they wanted the riders to remember why they were doing this. They wanted us to feel just a little more pain. Instead of continuing straight into town, after crossing into the town limits of Province-town, there was a little detour. It headed into Provincelands, where the dunes are the biggest on the Cape. There were three (you can be sure I counted) major hills left for us to conquer before we reached our goal. Some people had had it and started walking. I, of course, had to gut it out. There was nothing left in my leg. I had to segregate the pain to some other part of my brain and use all my will power to make it up those last few hills. I had no choice. That lack of choice helped. Failure was not an option. I was not going to take a sag wagon when I was within two miles of finishing. I had to go so slowly it was hard to keep the bike upright, but I pedaled up those damn dunes swearing at them on each pedal stroke. After number three, it really was all over. It was table flat. No need to go fast any more. I had made it.

Carole was a volunteer at the finish line. She took the ferry from Boston that morning to work the food tent. We all ate like pigs. She was going to work until our ferry back to Boston was ready to leave. After a shower, we loaded my bike onto the truck. I felt very self-satisfied, and it wasn't just the endorphins rushing through my bloodstream. I had raised a lot of money. I had worked hard since early spring to build up the kind of endurance I never knew I had. I had received comments from hundreds of people along the way. I had motivated some riders to stop whining and just do it. Best of all, the PMC money would go to the kind of research and treatment that had directly saved my life.

The fundraising events I participated in allowed me—no, made me—look outside myself to realize that my accomplishments not only raised money, but also inspired people. I thought I could and should do more. I remembered vividly what it felt like, as a sixteen-year-old, to lose a leg. I wanted to be able to share what I now know and feel with today's sixteen-year-olds. Andy, from the AIDS rides, was a teacher. He wanted his kids to hear my story. He arranged for me to speak to a room full of 150 sixteen-year-olds in Topsfield, Massachusetts. I followed a speech by Dan Kindlon, the Harvard psychologist and author of the books *Raising Cain: Protecting the Emotional Life of Boys* and *Too Much of a Good Thing: Raising Children of Character in an Indulgent Age*. That was a little intimidating. Dan was a great speaker who focused on the emotional life of boys and how it is threatened in modern society.

I started my speech with my leg on in business casual attire. I had a PowerPoint presentation ostensibly about self-esteem. I quickly achieved my goal of boring them. Before it got too bad, I had Andy come back up for a little improvised segue to the next part of my talk. He explained how we met and why we did the AIDS rides. While Andy spoke, I disappeared behind a screen and took off my leg and got into a pair of shorts.

I came back out, on crutches, carrying a jump rope. That immediately got their attention. *What was I going to do now?* I started jumping rope. First, I just jumped normally (but on one leg). Then I started doing crossovers, where my hands went from their respective sides of my body holding the rope handles to cross over in front of me. With experience—of which I had lots—I smoothly crossed my hands over and back in a semi-circular motion while the rope continued to smoothly travel its trajectory. It's just a simple feat of coordination, but it takes practice. While I was jumping, I asked the boys if any of them liked to jump rope. It's still an activity that girls do more than boys, but they had all seen Sylvester Stallone jumping rope in the Rocky movies at a frantic pace to get in shape for boxing. As a few of the boys tentatively raised their hands, I switched to backwards jumping.

My next question to them was, "Well, how many of you can jump on one leg?"

No hands up. "How many can jump one-legged and do crossovers?"

No hands. "How about backwards jumping with crossovers on one leg?"

Still no hands. Finally I said, "Okay, and what about backwards jumping with crossovers on one leg doing double jumps." I proceeded to switch to jumping really high and twirling the crossed-over rope around twice before I again hit the ground. By now, I had to stop or I would be out of breath for the entire time I was supposed to talk.

The point was not to show off (although that was a little fun, too), but to get their attention. When they first saw me legless, they were all shocked. They had probably not noticed my limp when I had my leg on. Their first reaction was to focus on the disability. *Gee, too bad this guy is disabled and probably can't do a lot of the cool stuff that I can do.* Before that thought was burned into any of their neurons, I was double jumping, crossed over and rock steady, on one leg. So the seed of doubt began to enter their minds. Now it was time for them to consider my initial premise: "What does any of this have to do with self-esteem?"

Once I caught my breath, I started to explain what had happened to me. How I had lost my leg. That it had happened when I was sixteen, just like them. "How would you handle it," I asked, "if it were you or one of your close friends? Would you visit your stricken friend in the hospital? Would you be afraid? Would you know how to help that friend overcome the shock of being disabled?" I was forcing them to imagine the unimaginable. I linked my disability, for which they were initially feeling pity, to a major blow to self-esteem. I linked my simple demonstration of tackling the physical challenge of one-legged rope jumping to gaining back lost self-esteem. I told them stories of skiing, whitewater rafting, waterskiing, long-distance bike riding, and swimming across San Francisco Bay to get them to place disabilities in a new light.

I was trying to shed a light on the difference between empathy and sympathy; the difference is important. While sympathy is the sharing in someone's pain—and it is a genuine and compassionate feeling—it can sometimes feel to the recipient like pity. Empathy, on the other hand, is identifying and trying to truly understand what someone is going through. If these teenagers could understand what it was like to have a disability, perhaps they wouldn't be as afraid of it. And just as important, they would be better prepared to deal with it themselves, if necessary, and more apt to know how to relate to others in that situation.

Mine ended up not being a weak presentation juxtaposed to that of Dan Kindlon, as I had feared it would be. They liked my talk and asked a lot of questions. Dan liked my talk, too, and put my story in his book *Too Much of a Good Thing*. At the end of my presentation, as I was putting away my props, I turned around to find a line of boys waiting to shake my hand. Their teachers hadn't put them up to this. It was spontaneous and natural. I was moved to tears. I might have had an impact on them after all. Knowing how hard that is to do with boys of that age made their gesture all the more gratifying.

Carole was impressed by the PMC ride, too. She saw the boundless energy and enthusiasm in all us committed riders, even though she was working the finish line where we were all at our lowest energy level. She saw how effective we could be at fundraising. She wanted to do the whole ride and not just serve food. Come spring, Carole wanted to train for her first ever long multi-day ride. I was thrilled, but nervous. On our first few training rides Carole was certain she was holding me back. She was right part of the time, but she was getting faster, stronger, and gaining endurance. I was happy to be patient. Riding alone gets old, and doing something I loved with her would be fantastic.

The next spring we started training as early as New England would let us. Snow lingered late, and then cold rains followed. Finally, by May, we were out a lot. Carole did not want the pressure of riding with me at first, so she did many of her own rides. She wisely wanted to ease into it. She had had knee twinges on some fun rides the previous season and wanted to avoid that pain. We did some rides together. I had to hold back to keep pace with her, but if I got into the right mindset, it was no problem. I knew I could always get in a high-intensity ride another day.

The day of the PMC came. Carole planned to do the full ride starting out in Sturbridge with me. Joanna drove us out and dropped us off before dawn. The only way back now was by bike. We started together, and I agreed that we would ride together as much as possible. If I forged ahead, I would always sync up with her at the very next water stop. That worked out, but I got antsy waiting at each rest stop; when she arrived, she never got enough rest. I was bad. It was a strange turn of events that the one-legged guy was riding harder and longer than the two-legged rider. I should have been getting used to that by now, but I wasn't. Her knee started to hurt a little the first day, but she made it to the Cape Cod Canal. She was not happy, but she was relieved. A shower and free beer helped a lot. Sleeping in a tent on the ground did not. It was the best option for us to be able to stay together. She was tense and nervous. It was impossible for her to enjoy the event. She did not sleep much, and reveille found her already awake. The ride on the Cape was misery for her. Her knee hurt so much that with every pedal stroke she chanted to herself, "I hate Jothy." We kept to the plan of syncing up at water stops, but it aggravated her all the same that I was not riding with her like I should have been. We made it to Provincetown with Carole in agony and me feeling a mixture of guilt that she was in pain and I hadn't always stayed with her, elation to have finished the ride again, and joy to have shared the experience after so many years of doing it without her.

Carole is a swimmer, too. She loves Walden Pond. When we were not training for the PMC, we enjoyed riding the twelve miles to Walden Pond where we would swim for a while before riding home. At first when I did these rides, I strapped crutches to the bike, locked the bike to a rack, and walked over to the water on crutches. Soon I realized I could hop down the five stairs to the sand with my bike and just lean it against the stone wall where we put our stuff while we swam. My bike is hard to steal since it has no right pedal, and the prospective thief would be pretty disappointed when he got on and tried to ride away.

Walden is an amazing place: a sanctuary amidst busy roads and the towns of Lincoln and Concord. When I reach the end of the pond and am halfway through my swim, I love standing on the bottom for a few seconds of rest listening to the quiet. The only sounds are the birds and maybe some splish-splashing from a nearby swimmer. The quiet and the solitude are very calming and healing.

Weston, a little town next to Newton, is on all my bike routes. It is the richest town in Massachusetts. The lots are big; houses are big; cars are big. The town center has angled parking along the street for stopping at the many shops sprinkled along the main drag. I always worry about riding past parked cars. There is the opening door threat, the sudden exit from a parking spot threat, and the pedestrian threat. I ride very cautiously; if I see an angled car starting to back up, I have time to either get quickly past it or stop well in advance of it moving into the street.

But my caution and ability to react in time assume one thing: sane drivers. On one particular ride through town, the driver of a huge Land Rover decided to hit it hard while backing up. I had no time to do either of my evasive maneuvers. I swerved, but he was moving so fast I put out my hand to push off of him. All that did was launch me off my bike into the middle of the road. Good thing this was a slow street and there was no oncoming traffic. I landed hard on my solar plexus. I had the wind resoundingly knocked out of me. I could not catch my breath. Luckily, the driver heard the noise and stopped before he crushed my bike or me. He quickly got out of his car to see what had happened. He saw my lack of a leg and frantically started looking under the back of the Land Rover for a missing appendage. It must not have occurred to him that a recently severed leg might be bleeding. Nor did it occur to him that I would not have sewed up pants covering my stump if the leg had just come off. I still could not breathe, much less talk, so I could not disabuse him of his certainty that his too-big vehicle that had backed up too fast had amputated my right leg. I just gestured to him and another bystander to come over and help me out of the middle of the street.

Sitting by the side of the street, I finally started to breathe and talk. He was much relieved to learn that my lost leg was not pinned up under his rear axle. Being in the center of Weston, we were right next to the fire and police station, and those guys must have been bored. I was quickly assigned an ambulance, police cruiser, and fire engine. They were desperate to do something—anything—for me. I would not go to the hospital, and they confirmed there was nothing structurally wrong with me. But I did let them put a band-aid on my scraped knee. Although I would feel the pain of bruised ribs for several weeks, I had escaped relatively unscathed.

Early in the spring of the second year I planned to do the Pan-Mass Challenge, the creator and director of the ride, Billy Starr, contacted me. He wanted to know if I would be the speaker at the event's kickoff. Riders who raised twice the minimum required to participate were called Heavy Hitters. This was a lot of money, since the minimum raise had climbed to over $4,200. Some Heavy Hitters were Extremely Rich Hitters and went way over the amount to qualify as Heavy. I was comfortably, but not excessively, Heavy, having raised more than $10,000 (all in relatively small donations of $100 or so). Billy grilled me about what I would say and what my theme might be. He must have liked what he heard because I got the job. I was thrilled. I love speaking in public. I love talking about my story. The PMC is a great cause, and it was a huge honor to be singled out to be the keynote speaker in front of such a high-powered audience. People kept telling me how great and motivating previous speakers had been. That set the bar high and made me nervous, but I was confident I could pull it off. When I am creating a speech, whether it's a toast at a family event or a public talk in front of hundreds, I don't share it with my family ahead of time if they are going to be in the audience. Carole and Joanna would be there, and I wanted their unaltered natural reaction.

The kickoff event was at the federal courthouse in Boston. There were TV cameras and bright lights. People sat at dinner tables. I had asked David Fialkow to introduce me. Dave was a venture partner at a VC firm I knew. He was on the board of directors of the PMC and a major participant in the ride. He was also a wild man, as I learned skiing with him in Utah the previous February. He got up at 4 a.m. to hike up the mountain at Alta on snowshoes. Dave had long hair combed straight back, was in constant motion, and always seemed distracted. He got to the dinner just in time to make the introduction. It was an impromptu speech. (Dave never prepares anything.) He referred to me as a hero. After all those years, I still couldn't quite come to terms with my effect on people. It still amazed me that when I told my story, people seemed to find inspiration in it. I walked up to that podium and told it again. I told them the frightening bits as well as the funny bits. The challenges as well as the successes. I received a standing ovation, but it was the look of pride and approval in Carole's and Joanna's eyes—where I looked to calibrate how I was doing during the talk—that made me choke up with pride and happiness.

After the difficulty she had during her first PMC ride, Carole figured she might do better with a new bike. She was more than correct. It was a dramatic transformation. Her new bike changed everything. Suddenly she rode at my speed. Her knee was no longer sore. Our training rides took on a whole new feel. At one point, while riding along at a natural pace for me, I turned my head to see that Carole was my wing mate right on my rear wheel. No longer was I riding at a slower pace than I really wanted to and occasionally feeling frustrated. Whether it was fifteen, thirty, or forty-five miles, she was now able to be a constant riding companion. It was clearly a whole lot more fun for her, too. She had signed up for the PMC ride again because she loved the cause and the experience, but she had been dreading the pain of the ride itself. She was going to train harder to try to be better prepared. Certainly, the extra training helped, but the bike helped most. Two people from work joined us on the ride; we formed our own little peloton. Carole never faltered and had a great ride.

Perhaps it was just in their honor since they were within earshot, but that year I received the strangest comments. "Best looking leg on the ride" and "great calf muscle" were my personal favorites. It made me wonder if at times women might like being objectified just a little. I really didn't mind it a bit. Carole's all time favorite was "Bobby Kennedy used to be my hero, but you just took his place." Pam's favorite was actually aimed at her: "Shame on you for drafting off of him," when she was exhausted and hanging on by riding in my slipstream.

Still, they got sick and tired of comment after comment directed at me. They later said to me, "Did they not see us? Are we chopped liver or what?" They threatened to get "I'm with Jothy" T-shirts made up for the next ride so they wouldn't feel left out.

Once I finally figured out that some things I say or do affect people in a positive way, it occurred to me that I should keep trying to reach a larger number of people. The fundraising bike rides became addictive. Giving talks to school kids became a rush. Everyone can relate to serious life challenges. I found myself wanting to do whatever I could to explain how I fought back from my challenges to become not only completely healthy, but to thrive.

Everyone gets hit with the "considering" epithet in some way for some thing. It stings, whether it's because you are too Black, too Asian, too female, too old, too young, or too disabled to perform in the manner in which some people think you are supposed to perform. People look for role models to follow so that they can break out of whatever constrains them. Whatever limits them. Whatever labels them. My story, my activities, my examples have in some way been an inspiration to some people. It took thirty years for me to begin to understand that I could have this impact.

When I get feeling too good about myself, just when I start losing any semblance of humility, it is friends and family that bring me back to reality. To them I am not an inspiration; I am just a friend, father, husband who happens to have one leg. But when my kids get serious, they express emotions that bring me the most satisfaction any father—or any one—can have. To hear my kids say they admire and respect me is the greatest accomplishment I can achieve in life. When I find they use me as an example in personal character statements or the subject of college application essays, I am moved to tears of pride, joy, and satisfaction.

With focus, drive, and determination, I have changed the nature of my disability. Some would say I have made it a *super*ability. This comes out in statements like, "I'll ride with the group, but don't expect me to keep up with Jothy," or "I'd love to go skiing with you guys, but I won't ski the runs Jothy skis," or "Sure, I'll swim Alcatraz, but don't expect me to be in Jothy's group of finishers." It's strange, but now when people talk about me as if I am abnormal, it is in the opposite way I once feared.

In swimming, people talk about the distances and times they can do, comparing themselves to each other, but leaving me out of it. Not because I'm slower, but because I'm faster. I'm faster only because I am determined. My determination is what makes me different, not my disability. It's almost as if "considering" has been turned around: "I'll finish after Jothy, considering I have two legs."

What is all too quickly forgotten is that I have to work harder than my able-bodied compatriots at whatever I do. Each year, getting ready for skiing, swimming, or biking is so much harder for me than for two-leggers (and two-lungers). By the time I am ready, others see only the results of all the pain and sweat. They put me off to the side in a separate category because I can do things most cannot do or will not attempt. And I can do them because I am willing to put up with more pain, and do more work, to get to where I want to go.

Determination and motivation are great equalizers for us all.

They can overcome the disadvantages of almost any disability, in much the same way that someone more determined and motivated is probably a better worker than someone who is not as determined, but has higher test scores and a better GPA. I believe it is true that I would not have accomplished as much in life—not just in athletics—if I had not lost a leg and a lung and had the threat of death hanging over me. Those experiences focused me, motivated me, and made me more determined than I might have been otherwise.

Others see my performance and accomplishments and forget, or can't imagine, what daily life is like for me. With all the skiing, mountain hiking, biking, and swimming, the idea that I can sometimes feel very disabled—even downright crippled—is foreign to many people who know me. This unpredictable range of emotion is a common phenomenon for someone with a disability, and the dependency on a prosthesis, or device of some kind, contributes to it.

My prosthesis is never for sports. It's for work, shopping, going out. It's nice not to be or look different all the time. Those are the times when different has to be on a completely dissimilar basis than through a perceived handicap. At work it needs to be solely on merit. Not having a leg that allows you to look and feel "normal" means the playing field is not level, and judgment will not be on merit alone, as it should be. I never want to be legless for important business meetings because of this. If it means I will elicit sympathy, then that is decidedly unwanted and unhelpful sympathy, which gets in the way of dealing with colleagues, employees, or outsiders. Even if there is no overt sympathy, reaching for crutches, hopping on one foot, even badly limping, it leaves me with a psychological feeling of an un-level playing field. This is why, after polio struck him, Fraklin Delano Roosevelt did not want to be seen in public in his wheelchair. When negotiating at Yalta, he wanted to be seated at the table first before the others came in because, in the climate of that day, he feared he would appear weak.

So regardless if my prosthesis is fitting or working poorly, my normal confidence, built up over time based on being able to ambulate—walk vertically—is suddenly challenged. The change from confident "normal" to insecure "invalid" can be very swift indeed. I remember walking out of a bar with a friend (sober) one evening, and tripping and falling. Immediately, a wave of bad feelings about the leg—and how it was able to instantly transform a carefree moment—washed over me. This is why the prosthesis should not just be thought of as a piece of medical equipment to support ambulation. It is a piece of psychological equipment of much more importance: it supports self-confidence.

If it hurts, I avoid getting up at a restaurant even to use the restroom. If it's not fitting, and I swear it's going to come off or at least make me stumble, I avoid going places. If I'm walking poorly or it's tiring to walk, I just do without whatever it was I would have gone to get. These feelings are relentless and insidious. They eat away at my self-confidence—even though I've had a prosthesis for thirty-five years. I constantly need a way to fight back. For me, taking the damn thing off and competing in a sport is one way. Working hard to get equipment that really works is another. The difference between the best technology and the basic leg is more than $35,000. That makes it completely inaccessible for most people around the world.

Even with a great leg, the feeling of disability can ebb and flow. The best technology still can't power the knee like a real one (yet). So, for me, walking up a hill is clumsy and tiring. No fit of plastic against skin is completely comfortable, so it hurts when I wear it for a long time. On uneven ground, I am clumsy. In tight places where the computer knee cannot detect normal unweighting, it acts like a peg leg, and I feel different all over again.

With poor technology or a poor fit, the leg can easily become unstable and unsafe. There is nothing like a few falls to leave me feeling insecure and disabled. Once I don't trust the leg, I walk stiff-legged with my hand in my pocket to help stabilize. Regaining lost trust after a nasty fall can take weeks.

Everything becomes difficult with a bad leg. I can't carry things. I can't walk any distance for lunch with colleagues or to catch a cab. I walk very slowly and laboriously through airports. I worry about just walking down the hall to my boss's office. It eats away at job effectiveness. It can affect how well I do my job, how likely a job promotion is, and therefore how much money I make. It affects my self-confidence in social relationships. I have trouble going over to visit friends for dinner, traveling to visit family or to go on vacation. Dealing with the superficiality of the disability is important for self-confidence. Dealing with the anatomic, physical, structural, mechanical aspects of the disability is just as important for success. With these daily challenges to self-confidence and self-esteem, the disabled person needs a constant outlet where they can excel, where they can overcompensate, where they can leave the temporarily able-bodied people in the dust.

Stories like mine are repeated thousands of times throughout the population. In many cases, the stories are much more compelling and impressive than mine. I wrote a book on debuggers because I had to work on a debugger and couldn't find anything written to help me understand how. After I figured it out, I wanted to save the next poor guy from having to go through that. I wrote a book about Internet security because my company needed to explain those concepts to people and nothing yet had been written that explained it well enough. So I figured it out myself.

As a sixteen-year-old lying in a hospital bed with one leg gone, with a mind on fire with anguish about how I might live a normal life, and then as a nineteen-year-old with one lung trying to recover from chemotherapy and deal with a death sentence, I felt on my own. I was looking for inspiration, guidance, motivation—anything. I wrote this book because I want to help anyone facing a disability or serious life trauma deal with it better and faster than I did. Considering it took me thirty years to figure it out well enough to be able to write it down, I hope my experiences can shorten the learning curve for someone in a similar situation. I will have succeeded if this book can provide someone who feels challenged by life the motivation to fight back to have what those polio survivors had: the drive and the will to compensate and then over-compensate. Not just physically, but in all aspects of life.

I've learned that people will forget what you said; people will forget what you did; but people will never forget how you made them feel.

— Maya Angelou, poet

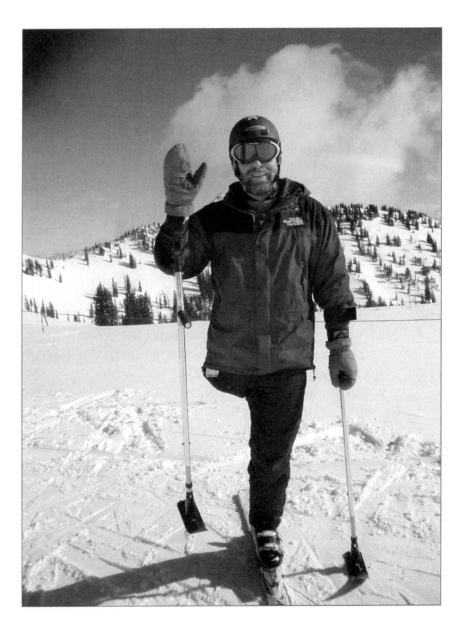

ABOUT THE AUTHOR

Jothy Rosenberg, north of 50 by a little bit, is an above-knee amputee caused by osteosarcoma in 1973. Three years later, the cancer metastasized and 2/5 of his lungs had to be removed. A course of chemotherapy—only just out in clinical use in 1976—is probably why he is still here today. He went on to get a PhD in computer science, be on the faculty of Duke University for five years, to author two technical books, to found seven high-tech companies, to ride in the Pan-Massachusetts Challenge bike-a-thon supporting the Dana-Farber Cancer Institute seven times, and to swim sixteen times from Alcatraz to San Francisco to support the Boston Healthcare for the Homeless Program. All told, his athletic fundraising efforts to date have netted the charities over $100,000. Jothy has a wonderful wife, three kids, a grandson, and a multitude of golden retrievers. He lives (and swims, and bikes) in Newton, Massachusetts. He wrote this book to try to share what he learned from thirty-five years living as a cancer survivor and an amputee, as someone who has recovered from very intense life trauma, in the hope it accelerates that learning for those in a similar situation and perhaps motivates and inspires those just needing a little lift.

A portion of the proceeds from this book go to the O'Brien Osteosarcoma fund at the Dana-Farber Cancer Institute in Boston.